A Culinary Journey to Vibrant Wellbeing: Heart Healthy Cookbook for Beginners:

Experience the Pleasure of Heart-Conscious Cooking for Everything from Breakfast to Special Occasions.

Alexandra Morgan

© 2023. All rights reserved.

Any content in this book may not be duplicated, reproduced, or transmitted in any way without the written permission of the publisher and author. The publisher and author disclaim all liability for any financial losses or damages, whether direct or indirect, that result from using or misusing the information in this publication.

Legal Advice: The copyright legislation protects this literature. The buyer may only use the content for personal purposes. Any part of this work reproduced, altered, sold, quoted, or distributed without permission in writing from the publisher or author is prohibited.

Note of caution: The content in this book is intended solely for illustrative and instructional purposes. Although every attempt has been made to guarantee timeliness, accuracy, and completeness, no warranties are offered. Readers should note that the author is not offering expert advice in any particular field, be it legal, financial, medical, or otherwise. This content has been compiled from several sources. You should seek advice from a licensed practitioner in the appropriate field before undertaking any of the methods outlined in this publication.

By using this content, readers agree that the author will not be held liable for any unfavorable results—losses or damages—that arise from using or interpreting the information—including any errors or omissions—provided.

TABLE OF CONTENTS

INTRODUCTION 7

The Significance of Heart Health 7

How to Use the Cookbook 7

Recognizing Heart Health 8

Macronutrient Balancing: The Basis for Heart Health 9

CHAPTER 1: BREAKFAST BOOSTERS 11

1.1 Nutty Banana Oat Pancakes 12

1.2 Avocado Sunrise Breakfast Wrap 13

1.3 Mediterranean Egg Muffins 14

1.4 Quinoa and Fruit Breakfast Parfait 15

1.5 Chia Seed Pudding with Mixed Berries 16

1.6 Spinach and Feta Omelet Roll 17

1.7 Blueberry Protein Pancakes 18

1.8 Greek Yogurt and Honey Granola Bowl 19

1.9 Tropical Mango Coconut Smoothie 20

1.10 Smoked Salmon and Avocado Bagel Stack 21

1.11 Cinnamon Apple Overnight Oats 22

CHAPTER 2: FRESH AND VIBRANT SALADS 23

2.1 Kale and Quinoa Power Salad with Lemon Vinaigrette 24

2.2 Pomegranate and Walnut Arugula Salad 25

2.3 Citrus Bliss Salad with Mixed Greens and Oranges 26

2.4 Mediterranean Greek Salad with Feta and Kalamata Olives 27

2.5 Grilled Chicken Caesar Salad with Whole-grain Croutons 28

2.6 Watermelon and Feta Salad with Mint 29

2.7 Roasted Beet and Goat Cheese Salad with Balsamic Glaze 30

2.8 Caprese Salad with Heirloom Tomatoes and Basil 31

2.9 Spinach and Strawberry Salad with Poppy Seed Dressing 32

CHAPTER 3: WHOLESOME SOUPS 33

3.1 Moroccan Chickpea Stew with Cilantro Drizzle 34

3.2 Spinach and Orzo Lemon Drop Soup 35

3.3 Tomato Basil Harmony Soup with Whole Wheat Croutons 36

3.4 Minestrone Medley Soup with Garden Vegetables 37

3.5 Creamy Cauliflower and Leek Soup 38

3.6 Spicy Black Bean and Sweet Potato Soup 39

3.7 Chicken and Vegetable Broth Elixir 40

3.8 Lentil and Spinach Delight Soup 41

3.9 Butternut Squash and Apple Bisque 42

CHAPTER 4: LEAN PROTEINS 43

4.1 Grilled Lemon Herb Salmon 44

4.2 Turkey and Quinoa Stuffed Bell Peppers 45

4.3 Baked Chicken Breast with Herbed Yogurt Marinade 46

4.4 Seared Tuna Steaks with Sesame Soy Glaze 47

4.5 Citrus-Marinated Grilled Shrimp Skewers 48

4.6 Mediterranean Chicken Skewers with Tzatziki 49

4.7 Blackened Tilapia with Mango Salsa 50

4.8 Balsamic Glazed Chicken Thighs 51

4.9 Spicy Chickpea and Turkey Lettuce Wraps 52

CHAPTER 5: NUTRIENT-PACKED SIDES 53

5.1 Garlic Lemon Roasted Brussels Sprouts 54

5.2 Quinoa and Kale Stuffed Bell Peppers 55

5.3 Sweet Potato and Black Bean Skillet 56

5.4 Broccoli Almond Crunch Salad 57

5.5 Spinach and Mushroom Quiche with Whole Wheat Crust 58

5.6 Avocado Cilantro Lime Rice 59

5.7 Roasted Asparagus with Parmesan and Lemon 60

5.8 Cauliflower and Chickpea Curry 61

5.9 Mediterranean Couscous Salad 62

CHAPTER 6: WHOLE-GRAIN WONDERS 63

6.1 Farro Salad with Roasted Vegetables and Feta 64

6.2 Quinoa and Black Bean Stuffed Peppers 65

6.3 Brown Rice and Vegetable Stir-Fry 66

6.4 Whole Wheat Mediterranean Pizza with Hummus Base 67

6.5 Spaghetti Squash Primavera 68

6.6 Whole-grain Couscous with Lemon and Herbs 69

6.7 Wild Rice Pilaf with Cranberries and Almonds 70

6.8 Bulgur and Chickpea Salad with Tahini Dressing 71

6.9 Oat and Chia Seed Breakfast Bowl 72

CHAPTER 7: SNACK ATTACK **73**

7.1 Trail Mix with Nuts and Dried Fruit 74

7.2 Guacamole with Baked Whole Wheat Tortilla Chips 75

7.3 Greek Yogurt and Berry Parfait 76

7.4 Apple Slices with Almond Butter and Cinnamon 77

7.5 Cottage Cheese and Pineapple Kabobs 77

7.6 Spiced Roasted Chickpeas 78

7.7 Dark Chocolate-Dipped Strawberries 79

7.8 Avocado and Tomato Salsa 80

7.9 Hummus-Stuffed Mini Bell Peppers 81

CHAPTER 8: SWEET INDULGENCES **82**

8.1 Dark Chocolate Avocado Mousse 83

8.2 Berry and Yogurt Parfait with Honey Drizzle 84

8.3 Baked Apples with Cinnamon and Walnuts 85

8.4 Mango Coconut Chia Pudding 86

8.5 Banana-Oatmeal Cookies with Raisins 87

8.6 Almond Butter Banana Ice Cream 88

8.7 Greek Yogurt Berry Popsicles 89

8.8 Chocolate-Dipped Strawberries with Pistachios 90

8.9 Raspberry Lemon Sorbet 91

8.10 Pumpkin Spice Energy Bites 92

CHAPTER 9: HYDRATION STATION **93**

9.1 Citrus Burst Infused Water 94

9.2 Berry Bliss Hydration Elixir 95

9.3 Minty Cucumber Spa Quencher 96

9.4 Green Tea and Berry Fusion 97

9.5 Watermelon Mint Cooler 98

CHAPTER 10: COOKING BASICS FOR BEGINNERS 99

10.1 Easy Pan-Seared Chicken Breast 100

10.2 Simple Spaghetti Bolognese 101

10.3 Roasted Vegetables with Olive Oil and Herbs 102

10.4 Classic Tomato Basil Pasta Sauce 103

10.5 Fluffy Scrambled Eggs with Herbs 104

10.6 Perfectly Steamed Broccoli 105

10.7 Homemade Chicken Noodle Soup 106

10.8 Basic Baked Salmon Fillets 107

10.9 Creamy Mashed Potatoes 108

10.10 Sautéed Garlic Shrimp 109

CHAPTER 11: CELEBRATING SPECIAL OCCASIONS 110

11.1 Elegant Shrimp Cocktail Platter 110

11.2 Herb-Crusted Prime Rib Roast 111

11.3 Decadent Chocolate Ganache Cake 112

11.10 Smoked Salmon and Caviar Canapés 113

11.4 Sparkling Pomegranate Champagne Punch 114

11.5 Lobster Tail Thermidor 115

11.6 Truffle-Infused Wild Mushroom Risotto 116

11.7 Citrus-Glazed Herb-Roasted Turkey 117

11.8 Caramelized Onion and Gruyère Tartlets 118

11.9 Grand Marnier Soufflé with Vanilla Sauce 119

CONCLUSION 120

INDEX 121

INTRODUCTION

Greetings and salutations from the "Heart Healthy Cookbook for Beginners"—the starting point for a delectable journey towards better heart health! This cookbook is made with you in mind, whether you're new to heart-conscious cooking or looking for new ideas to keep your cardiovascular health in check.

It is more important than ever to prioritize heart health in today's fast-paced world. This cookbook attempts to make the journey toward heart-healthy living pleasurable and attainable, particularly for individuals new to cooking. We firmly believe that a heart-healthy lifestyle begins in the kitchen.

The Significance of Heart Health

Allow me to explain the importance of heart health before starting with the recipes. Your body's engine, your heart, depends heavily on the sustenance you eat to maintain optimal heart health. A heart-healthy diet can help people live longer, more active lives, reduce their risk of cardiovascular illnesses, and improve their general well-being.

How to Use the Cookbook

This cookbook offers a guide to making delicious, low-fat meals without sacrificing flavor—it's more than just a collection of recipes. You will find various recipes on these pages for breakfast, lunch, dinner, snacks, and even special events. Each dish has been carefully crafted to be as simple as possible, making it suitable for inexperienced and seasoned cooks.

Educational Insights: You'll find tidbits of nutritional knowledge, advice on heart-healthy cooking methods, and details on the essential components that support cardiovascular health throughout the book. Not only do we want to give you recipes, but we also want to arm you with information that will motivate you to lead a heart-healthy lifestyle in the long run.

A Visual Delight: Get ready to be amazed by the sights! Each recipe comes with scrumptious photos that give you an idea of the delicious foods waiting to be prepared in your kitchen. We think a gorgeous presentation makes the food taste better overall and motivates you to savor your heart-healthy dishes.

Alright, let's get started:

Set out on this gastronomic adventure with assurance, knowing that every recipe has been painstakingly chosen to please your palate and uplift your spirits. Whether you're preparing food for your loved ones, yourself, or friends, these recipes are meant to make eating heart-healthy a fun and sustainable life choice.

We appreciative that you selected the "Heart Healthy Cookbook for Beginners." May you be joyful when you smell meals that not only tantalize your taste senses but also support heart health and hear the sounds of beneficial ingredients sizzling in your kitchen.

Cheers to tasty and heart-healthy food!

Recognizing Heart Health

Here, we explore the fundamentals of heart health at the center of our gastronomic adventure. Prioritizing heart health is an important and fulfilling undertaking. Let's discuss this before diving into the delectable recipes in this cookbook.

The Value of a Diet Good for the Heart

A heart-healthy diet is a thread that weaves a story of resilience, vitality, and well-being throughout our lives. The importance of eating a heart-healthy diet extends well beyond the avoidance of heart disease. It's a dedication to taking care of the most important organ in your body and, consequently, improving your quality of life.

Your Heart, the Keeper of Cardiovascular Wellness

Your heart is your body's constant protector, coordinating the flow of life throughout it. Maintaining a heart-healthy diet is an important gesture of support, recognizing this powerful organ's vital role in keeping life alive. You may extend the life and resiliency of your heart by eating foods that support cardiovascular health.

Lowering the Risk: Protecting Against Heart Diseases

Heart-related conditions, such as coronary artery disease and heart attacks, are the leading causes of death globally. A heart-healthy diet reduces risk factors, including obesity, high blood pressure, and cholesterol, like a strong shield. By choosing nutrient-dense foods and making thoughtful decisions, you actively protect your heart from possible threats.

Achieving Ideal Cholesterol Levels: A delicate balance

Despite its negative connotations, cholesterol has a complex relationship with heart health. The goal of a heart-healthy diet is to keep "good" (HDL) and "bad" (LDL) cholesterol levels in check. You may support optimal cardiac function by influencing this balance with well-chosen ingredients and cooking methods.

Harmony of Blood Pressure: Methods for Reducing Sodium

Your heart is put under unnecessary strain by high blood pressure. Reducing salt consumption is emphasized in a heart-healthy diet since it is a major cause of high blood pressure. You can make tasty, heart-healthy meals by embracing herbs and spices as flavoring agents and finding palatable substitutes.

Weight Control: A Heart-Healthy Partner

Maintaining a healthy weight is essential for heart health promotion. Weight management is facilitated by eating a diet high in whole, nutrient-dense foods and practicing portion control. As a result, your heart is under less stress and can beat more smoothly and effectively.

Beyond the Body: Welfare of the Mind and Spirit

Research on the relationship between heart-healthy eating and mental wellness is expanding. Nutrient-dense foods have been connected to improved mood, improved cognitive performance, and a decreased risk of mental health issues. Eating healthfully for your body also benefits your mind and spirit.

Developing cardiovascular fitness requires navigating a complex nutritional terrain, so following the Basic Nutrition Guidelines for Cardiovascular Fitness is so important. Our eating choices have a direct impact on the condition of our hearts. Together, let's set out on this adventure to learn the fundamental dietary recommendations that act as road signs for a heart-healthy way of living.

Macronutrient Balancing: The Basis for Heart Health

The careful balance of macronutrients, proteins, carbs, and fats is crucial to cardiovascular health. Lean proteins, complex carbs, and unsaturated fats should be prioritized in a heart-healthy diet, but consumption of saturated and trans fats should be controlled. This equilibrium supports ideal cardiac function and offers vital nutrients for general health.

Accepting High-Fibre Diets: Nature's Heart-Healing Agents

When it comes to heart health, fiber is an unsung hero. Fiber plentiful in whole grains, legumes, fruits, and vegetables, helps maintain a healthy digestive tract and lower cholesterol. Accept a vibrant range of plant-based foods to guarantee sufficient heart-healthy fibers.

The Fatty Acids Omega-3: Taking Care of Your Heart

Omega-3 fatty acids found in walnuts, flaxseeds, chia seeds, and fatty fish are essential for heart health. These necessary fats boost heart health generally, lower inflammation, and enhance cholesterol profiles. It's a tasty investment in your heart health to include foods high in omega-3s in your diet.

Conscientious Sodium Control: Maintaining Heart Equilibrium

Although the body needs sodium for proper functioning, too much can lead to hypertension and cardiac strain. Minimizing processed foods, selecting fresh ingredients, and experimenting with herbs and spices to boost flavor without overdoing the salt are all part of a heart-healthy diet.

Portion Control: A Heart-Centered Approach to Eating Moderation is fundamental in promoting cardiovascular wellness. Keeping an eye on portion sizes promotes weight control by lowering the risk of heart problems associated with obesity and helps prevent overconsumption of calories. Deliberately savoring every bite, you may respect your body's requirements and enjoy your meals.

Hydration: Heart Health's Elixir

Maintaining proper hydration is essential for heart health. Water is essential for maintaining blood volume, promoting the movement of nutrients, and sustaining all body functions. The best way to keep your heart hydrated is to limit your intake of sugar-filled drinks and stick to drinking water as your primary beverage.

Foods High in Antioxidants: Nature's Defense System

Vibrant fruits and vegetables are rich in antioxidants, which protect your heart by scavenging free radicals that can cause inflammation. Various antioxidants are provided by including a wide variety of colorful produce in your diet, which strengthens your heart's defenses against oxidative stress.

Nutritional Information (per serving):

Please note that the amounts and brands of certain products used may cause variations in the nutritional values shown. Use a nutrition calculator using the selected ingredients for precise information.

CHAPTER 1: BREAKFAST BOOSTERS

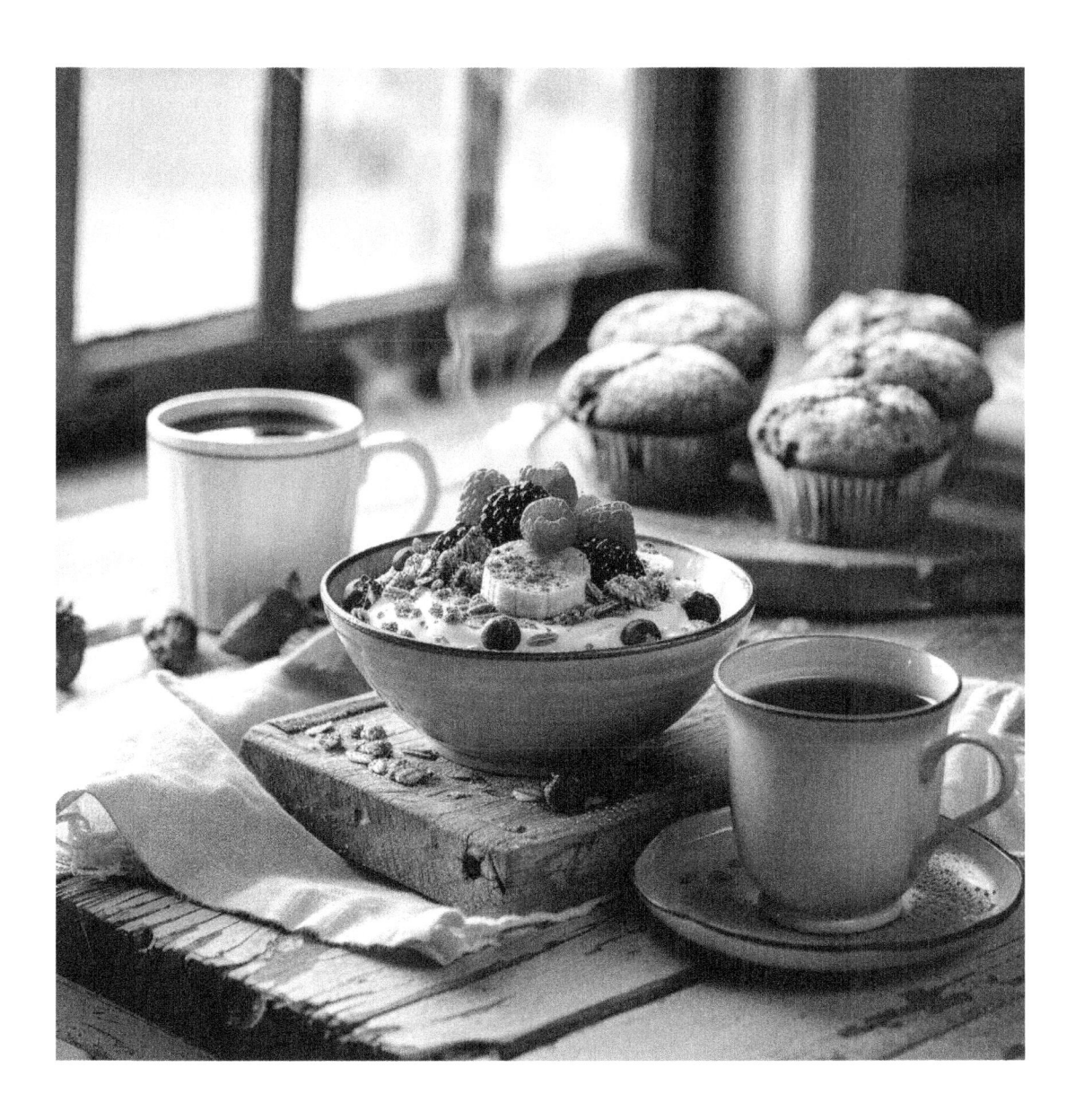

1.1 Nutty Banana Oat Pancakes

Preparation time	Cooking time	Servings
20 minutes	10-12 minutes	2

INGREDIENTS:

- 1 cup (90g) rolled oats
- 2 ripe bananas
- 2 large eggs
- 1/2 cup (120ml) milk (any type you prefer)
- 1/4 cup (30g) chopped nuts (such as walnuts or almonds)
- 1 teaspoon baking powder
- 1/2 teaspoon vanilla extract
- Pinch of salt
- Butter or cooking spray for the pan

INSTRUCTIONS:

1. Combine the rolled oats, ripe bananas, eggs, milk, chopped nuts, vanilla extract, baking powder, and a pinch of salt in a blender.
2. Blend the ingredients until the mixture is smooth and thoroughly combined.
3. Allow the batter to rest for approximately 5-10 minutes. This helps the oats absorb the liquid and gives you fluffier pancakes.
4. Heat a non-stick skillet or griddle over medium heat. Add a small amount of butter or cooking spray to coat the surface.
5. Pour 1/4 cup of batter onto the heated skillet for each pancake. Cook until bubbles form on top, flip and continue cooking until the other side is golden brown.
6. Repeat the process with the remaining batter, adjusting the heat as needed.
7. Stack the pancakes on plates and top with additional banana slices, a sprinkle of nuts, and a drizzle of maple syrup if desired.

Nutritional Information (per serving):

Calories: 629 | Fat: 20.7g | Saturated Fat: 5g | Cholesterol: 374mg | Sodium: 287mg | Carbohydrate: 88.5g | Fiber: 9.9g | Protein: 23.3g

NOTES:

- This recipe makes approximately 6-8 pancakes, depending on your preferred size.
- Personalize your toppings with fresh fruit, yogurt, or a dab of nut butter for extra taste.

1.2 Avocado Sunrise Breakfast Wrap

Preparation time	Cooking time	Servings
15 minutes	-	2

INGREDIENTS:

- 2 large whole-grain tortillas
- 2 large eggs
- 1 ripe avocado, sliced
- 1 medium tomato, diced (about 1 cup or 150g)
- 1/4 cup (40g) red onion, finely chopped
- Fresh cilantro, chopped (for garnish)
- Salt and pepper to taste
- Optional: Hot sauce or salsa for extra flavor

INSTRUCTIONS:

1. Slice the avocado, dice the tomato, and finely chop the red onion. Set aside.
2. Beat eggs in a bowl, adding a pinch of salt and pepper for seasoning.
3. Add the beaten eggs to a nonstick pan warmed over medium heat.
4. Scramble the eggs until thoroughly cooked, and then take them off the heat.
5. To make the tortillas malleable, place them in a dry pan or give them a quick 10 to 15 seconds in the microwave.
6. Arrange the warmed tortillas on a clean surface.
7. Divide the scrambled eggs equally between the two tortillas, placing them in the center.
8. Arrange the sliced avocado, diced tomatoes, and chopped red onion over the scrambled eggs.
9. Sprinkle fresh cilantro over the ingredients for added flavor and freshness.
10. Season with additional salt and pepper to taste.
11. Optional: Spoon salsa or drizzle with hot sauce over the filling if you want spicy food.
12. Fold the sides of the tortillas toward the center, creating a wrap.

Nutritional Information (per serving):

Calories: 534 | Fat: 26.2g | Saturated Fat: 7.8g | Cholesterol: 372mg | Sodium: 20109mg | Carbohydrate: 53.9g | Fiber: 12.6g | Protein: 24g

NOTES:

- Feel free to customize the fillings based on your preferences—additions like cheese, spinach, or bell peppers work well.
- For a well-rounded breakfast, think about serving with a small green salad or fresh fruit.

1.3 Mediterranean Egg Muffins

Preparation time	Cooking time	Servings
15 minutes	**15-18 minutes**	**2**

INGREDIENTS:

- 4 large eggs
- 1/4 cup (60ml) milk
- 1/2 cup (75g) cherry tomatoes, diced
- 1/4 cup (30g) feta cheese, crumbled
- 1/4 cup (40g) black olives, sliced
- 1/4 cup (30g) red onion, finely chopped
- 1 tablespoon (15ml) olive oil
- 1 teaspoon dried oregano
- Salt and pepper to taste
- Fresh parsley, chopped (for garnish)

INSTRUCTIONS:

1. Preheat your oven to 350°F (180°C).
2. Apply olive oil to the muffin tin for greasing or paper liners.
3. Whisk the eggs and milk together thoroughly in a bowl.
4. Stir in the diced cherry tomatoes, crumbled feta cheese, sliced black olives, finely chopped red onion, olive oil, dried oregano, salt, and pepper. Mix until ingredients are evenly distributed.
5. Fill each muffin tin cup to about two-thirds of the way to the top before dividing the egg mixture among them evenly.
6. Place the muffin pan in the oven that has been warmed, and bake for 15 to 18 minutes, or until the tops are golden brown and the eggs are set.
7. Give the egg muffins a few minutes to cool in the muffin tray. Garnish with chopped fresh parsley.

Nutritional Information (per serving):

Calories: 902 | Fat: 76g | Saturated Fat: 16.4g | Cholesterol: 756mg | Sodium: 544mg | Carbohydrate: 37.8g | Fiber: 22.4g | Protein: 33.3g

NOTES:

- Add spinach, sun-dried tomatoes, and your favorite Mediterranean ingredients to customize the recipe.
- Feel free to sprinkle extra feta cheese or herbs on top before baking for added flavor.

_____
_____
_____
_____

1.4 Quinoa and Fruit Breakfast Parfait

Preparation time	Cooking time	Servings
10 minutes	-	2

INGREDIENTS:

- 1/2 cup (90g) quinoa, cooked and cooled
- 1 cup (240g) Greek yogurt (unsweetened)
- 1 cup (150g) mixed fruits (such as berries, mango, and kiwi), diced
- 2 tablespoons (30g) nuts or seeds (e.g., almonds, chia seeds)
- 2 tablespoons (30ml) honey or maple syrup
- 1/2 teaspoon vanilla extract
- Fresh mint leaves for garnish (optional)

INSTRUCTIONS:

1. Cook the quinoa as per the directions provided on the package. Allow it to cool to room temperature.
2. Add the Greek yogurt, vanilla extract, and honey (or maple syrup) to a bowl. Mix well until smooth.
3. In serving glasses or bowls, begin by layering the bottom with a spoonful of cooked quinoa.
4. Spoon a layer of the sweetened Greek yogurt on top of the quinoa.
5. Add a layer of mixed fruits over the yogurt.
6. Sprinkle a portion of nuts or seeds on top.
7. Once the glass or bowl is full, continue layering until you reach the top, where you should place a layer of fruits and then scatter some nuts or seeds.
8. Optionally, garnish with fresh mint leaves for a burst of freshness.

Nutritional Information (per serving):

Calories: 1149 | Fat: 54.1g | Saturated Fat: 7.9g | Cholesterol: 3mg | Sodium: 694mg | Carbohydrate: 141.1g | Fiber: 11.9g | Protein: 26.9g

NOTES: Depending on your taste preferences, you can customize the sweetness by changing the honey or maple syrup.

_____
_____
_____
_____

1.5 Chia Seed Pudding with Mixed Berries

Preparation time	Cooking time	Servings
5 minutes	-	2

INGREDIENTS:

- 1/4 cup (48g) chia seeds
- 1 cup (240ml) unsweetened almond milk (or any milk of your choice)
- 1 tablespoon (15ml) maple syrup or honey (adjust to taste)
- 1/2 teaspoon vanilla extract
- a mixture of berries (strawberries, blueberries, raspberries) to use as a topping
- Optional: Sliced almonds or shredded coconut for garnish

INSTRUCTIONS:

1. Combine chia seeds, almond milk, maple syrup or honey, and vanilla extract in a bowl. To disperse the chia seeds equally, stir well.
2. Refrigerate the bowl for a minimum of three hours or overnight, covered. Over this period, the chia seeds will absorb the liquid, giving the mixture a pudding-like texture.
3. Before serving, thoroughly stir the chia seed pudding to break up clumps and ensure a smooth texture.
4. Spoon the chia seed pudding into serving glasses or bowls.
5. Arrange a generous amount of mixed berries on the chia seed pudding.
6. If desired, garnish with sliced almonds or shredded coconut for added texture.

Nutritional Information (per serving):

Calories: 271 | Fat: 4.7g | Saturated Fat: 0.5g | Cholesterol: 0mg | Sodium: 45mg | Carbohydrate: 42.4g | Fiber: 4.5g | Protein: 2.3g

NOTES: Feel free to customize the sweetness by adjusting the amount of maple syrup or honey.

1.6 Spinach and Feta Omelet Roll

Preparation time	Cooking time	Servings
10 minutes	12-15 minutes	2

INGREDIENTS:

- 4 large eggs
- 1/4 cup (60ml) milk
- 1 cup (30g) fresh spinach, chopped
- 1/4 cup (60g) feta cheese, crumbled
- 1/4 cup (30g) red bell pepper, diced
- 1/4 cup (30g) red onion, finely chopped
- Salt and pepper to taste
- Cooking spray or butter for greasing

INSTRUCTIONS:

1. Preheat your oven to 375°F (190°C).
2. Finely chop the red onion, dice the red bell pepper, crumble the feta cheese, and chop the fresh spinach.
3. Whisk the eggs and milk together thoroughly in a bowl. Add pepper and salt for seasoning.
4. Add the sliced red bell pepper, finely chopped red onion, crumbled feta cheese, and chopped spinach to the egg mixture.
5. Grease a baking sheet lightly with butter or cooking spray after lining it with parchment paper.
6. Scatter the egg mixture evenly to form a thin layer on the baking sheet that has been prepared.
7. Bake in a preheated oven for 12 to 15 minutes or until the omelet is set through and has a hint of color.
8. Once cooked, carefully roll the omelet from one end to the other while it's still warm.
9. Allow the omelet roll to cool slightly, then slice it into rounds. Serve warm.

Nutritional Information (per serving):

Calories: 474 | Fat: 24.7g | Saturated Fat: 8.7g | Cholesterol: 756mg | Sodium: 488mg | Carbohydrate: 39.2g | Fiber: 14.8g | Protein: 34.6g

NOTES: Customize the filling by adding cherry tomatoes, mushrooms, or herbs.

_____
_____
_____
_____

1.7 Blueberry Protein Pancakes

Preparation time	Cooking time	Servings
15 minutes	10-12 minutes	2

INGREDIENTS:

- 1 cup (90g) rolled oats
- 1 scoop (about 30g) vanilla protein powder
- 1 teaspoon baking powder
- 1/2 teaspoon cinnamon
- 1/2 cup (120ml) milk (any type you prefer)
- 1 large egg
- 1 tablespoon (15ml) maple syrup or honey
- 1 teaspoon vanilla extract
- 1/2 cup (75g) fresh or frozen blueberries
- Cooking spray or butter for greasing

INSTRUCTIONS:

1. Combine the rolled oats, vanilla protein powder, baking powder, cinnamon, milk, egg, maple syrup or honey, and vanilla extract. Blend until you have a smooth batter in a blender.
2. Incorporate the blueberries gently into the pancake batter by folding them in.
3. Heat a nonstick pan or grill to a medium temperature. Use butter or cooking spray to oil it lightly.
4. For every pancake, pour 1/4 cup of batter onto the hot griddle. Turn the pancakes over and cook the second side until golden brown, or cook for a few more minutes until surface bubbles appear. As a result, the pancakes will cook evenly and have a gorgeous golden finish.
5. Repeat the process until all the batter is used, adjusting the heat as needed.
6. Stack the pancakes on plates and serve them warm.

Nutritional Information (per serving):

Calories: 849 | Fat: 10.4g | Saturated Fat: 2.6g | Cholesterol: 206mg | Sodium: 247mg | Carbohydrate: 126.1g | Fiber: 20g | Protein: 55.5g

NOTES: Add more fresh blueberries, a dollop of Greek yogurt, or a drizzle of maple syrup to personalize your toppings.

_____
_____
_____
_____

1.8 Greek Yogurt and Honey Granola Bowl

Preparation time	Cooking time	Servings
5 minutes	-	2

INGREDIENTS:

- 2 cups (480g) Greek yogurt (unsweetened)
- 4 tablespoons (60g) honey
- 1 cup (100g) granola
- 1 cup (150g) mixed fresh berries (such as strawberries, blueberries, and raspberries)
- 2 tablespoons (30g) chopped nuts (e.g., almonds or walnuts)
- Optional: For added nourishment, mix in some flaxseeds or chia seeds.

INSTRUCTIONS:

1. In a bowl, scoop out the Greek yogurt as the base of your bowl.
2. Drizzle the honey over the Greek yogurt, adjusting the amount to your desired sweetness.
3. Sprinkle the granola evenly over the Greek yogurt for a crunchy texture.
4. Arrange the mixed fresh berries on top of the granola.
5. Sprinkle the chopped nuts over the berries for added crunch and flavor.
6. You can add a sprinkle of chia seeds or flaxseeds for extra nutrition.
7. Mix all the ingredients together, or enjoy the layers separately as you prefer.

Nutritional Information (per serving):

Calories: 1351 | Fat: 65.7g | Saturated Fat: 10.4g | Cholesterol: 5mg | Sodium: 723mg | Carbohydrate: 224.7g | Fiber: 14.9g | Protein: 35.8g

NOTES:

- Feel free to customize by adding your favorite fruits, such as banana slices or mango chunks.
- Experiment with different types of granola to vary the flavors and textures.

_____
_____
_____
_____

1.9 Tropical Mango Coconut Smoothie

Preparation time	Cooking time	Servings
10 minutes	-	2

INGREDIENTS:

- 2 cups (300g) frozen mango chunks
- 1 cup (240ml) coconut milk
- 1 cup (240ml) plain Greek yogurt
- 2 tablespoons (30g) shredded coconut (unsweetened)
- 2 tablespoons (30ml) honey or agave syrup (optional, depending on sweetness preference)
- Ice cubes (optional for extra chill)
- Garnish: Fresh mint leaves or additional shredded coconut

INSTRUCTIONS:

1. Blend the frozen mango chunks, Greek yogurt, shredded coconut, coconut milk, and honey (if desired) in a blender.
2. Blend until smooth and creamy.
3. You can adjust the smoothie's consistency by adding a small amount of extra coconut milk if it's too thick.
4. Pour a few ice cubes into the blender and process until completely combined for an additional cool touch.
5. Transfer the smoothie into a glass and decorate with shredded coconut or fresh mint leaves.

Nutritional Information (per serving):

Calories: 868 | Fat: 46.4g | Saturated Fat: 40.7g | Cholesterol: 4mg | Sodium: 55mg | Carbohydrate: 117.3g | Fiber: 11.9g | Protein: 10.7g

NOTES: If your mango is naturally sweet, reduce or eliminate the honey to customize the sweetness.

_____
_____
_____
_____

1.10 Smoked Salmon and Avocado Bagel Stack

Preparation time	Cooking time	Servings
15 minutes	-	2

(This recipe doesn't require cooking beyond toasting the bagel.)

INGREDIENTS:

- 2 whole-grain or everything bagels, sliced and toasted
- 4 oz (120g) smoked salmon
- 1 ripe avocado, thinly sliced
- 4 tablespoons (60g) cream cheese
- 2 tablespoons (30ml) capers, drained
- Fresh dill for garnish
- Lemon wedges for serving

INSTRUCTIONS:

1. Slice the bagel and toast it to your desired level of crispiness.
2. Spread the cream cheese evenly on both halves of the toasted bagel.
3. Arrange the thinly sliced avocado on top of the cream cheese.
4. Place the smoked salmon over the avocado, ensuring an even distribution.
5. Sprinkle the drained capers over the smoked salmon for a salty flavor.
6. Garnish the bagel stack with fresh dill for a touch of herbaceous aroma.
7. Serve the Smoked Salmon and Avocado Bagel Stack with lemon wedges on the side for a zesty finish.

Nutritional Information (per serving):

Calories: 1270 | Fat: 96.1g | Saturated Fat: 49.8g | Cholesterol: 452mg | Sodium: 7735mg | Carbohydrate: 47.4g | Fiber: 14.8g | Protein: 71.8g

NOTES:

- Experiment with different types of bagels for varied flavors.
- Feel free to add red onion slices or cherry tomatoes for extra freshness.

_____
_____
_____
_____

1.11 Cinnamon Apple Overnight Oats

Preparation time	Cooking time	Servings
5 minutes	-	2

INGREDIENTS:

- 1 cup (90g) rolled oats
- 1 cup (240ml) milk (dairy or plant-based)
- 1 cup (240g) Greek yogurt
- 1 apple, cored and diced
- 2 tablespoons (30ml) maple syrup or honey
- 1 teaspoon ground cinnamon
- 1/2 teaspoon vanilla extract
- Optional toppings: Sliced almonds, chopped walnuts, or additional diced apples

INSTRUCTIONS:

1. Place the rolled oats, milk, Greek yogurt, chopped apple, ground cinnamon, maple syrup, and vanilla essence in a jar or other lidded container.
2. Stir the ingredients until well combined, ensuring the oats are fully immersed in the liquid.
3. Refrigerate the jar or container for at least 4 hours or overnight, covered. As a result, the oats can soak and become softer.
4. Before serving, give the mixture a good stir to incorporate any settled ingredients.
5. If desired, top your Cinnamon Apple Overnight Oats with sliced almonds, chopped walnuts, or diced apples for extra texture and flavor.

Nutritional Information (per serving):

Calories: 767 | Fat: 6.3g | Saturated Fat: 2.2g | Cholesterol: 7mg | Sodium: 60mg | Carbohydrate: 164.3g | Fiber: 34.3g | Protein: 15.6g

NOTES:

- Depending on your taste preferences, change the amount of honey or maple syrup to change the sweetness.
- Feel free to experiment with different types of apples for varied textures and flavors.

_____
_____
_____
_____

CHAPTER 2: FRESH AND VIBRANT SALADS

These salads are nutritious but also bursting with colors and flavors to make your meals both satisfying and delightful. Enjoy the freshness!

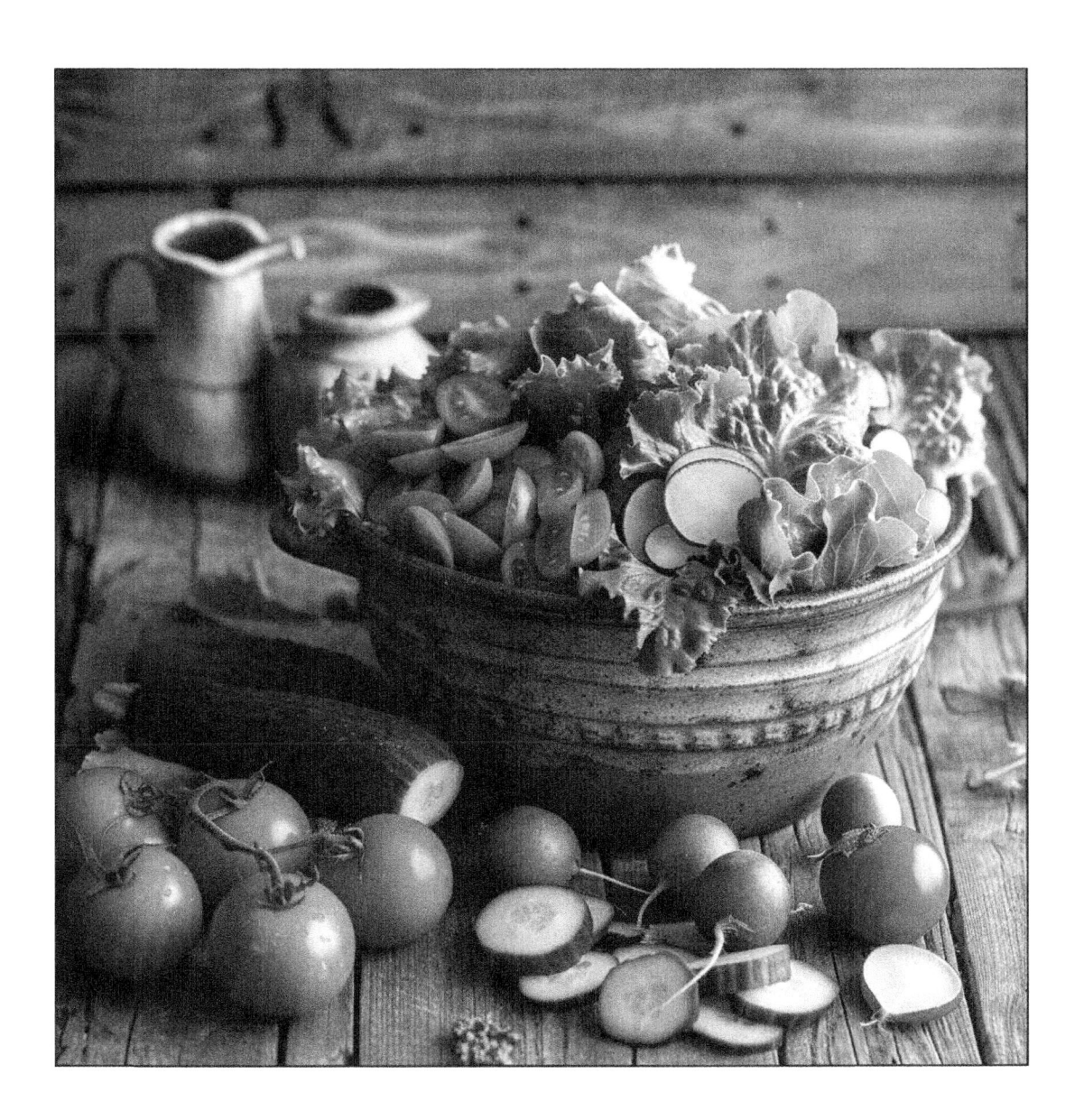

2.1 Kale and Quinoa Power Salad with Lemon Vinaigrette

Preparation time	Cooking time	Servings
20 minutes	15 minutes (is mainly for the quinoa)	2

INGREDIENTS:

For Salad:

- 2 cups (350g) cooked quinoa, cooled
- 4 cups (120g) kale, stems removed and finely chopped
- 1/2 cup (60g) cherry tomatoes, halved
- 1/2 cup (60g) cucumber, diced
- 1/2 cup (60g) red bell pepper, diced
- 4 tablespoons (30g) red onion, finely chopped
- 4 tablespoons (60g) feta cheese, crumbled
- 2 tablespoons (30g) pumpkin seeds (pepitas)

For Lemon Vinaigrette:

- 4 tablespoons (60ml) extra virgin olive oil
- 2 tablespoons (30ml) lemon juice
- 2 teaspoons honey
- 1 teaspoon Dijon mustard
- 2 cloves garlic, minced
- Salt and pepper to taste

INSTRUCTIONS:

For Kale and Quinoa Power Salad:

1. Prepare the quinoa and allow it to cool as directed on the package.
2. To soften the finely chopped kale, massage it in a big bowl for a few minutes with a small amount of olive oil.
3. Add cooled quinoa, cherry tomatoes, cucumber, red bell pepper, red onion, crumbled feta cheese, and pumpkin seeds to the bowl with kale.

For Lemon Vinaigrette (whisk or mix the ingredients well to combine them thoroughly):

1. Add the extra virgin olive oil, lemon juice, honey, Dijon mustard, minced garlic, salt, and pepper to a small bowl and mix well. Mix until well combined.
2. Taste the vinaigrette and adjust the seasoning according to your preference.
3. Drizzle the lemon vinaigrette over the salad.
4. Gently toss the salad to coat the ingredients with the vinaigrette evenly.
5. Serve the Kale and Quinoa Power Salad immediately, or refrigerate if chilled.

Nutritional Information (per serving):

Calories: 3872 | Fat: 286.4g | Saturated Fat: 67.5g | Cholesterol: 178mg | Sodium: 2983mg | Carbohydrate: 286.5g | Fiber: 36.6g | Protein: 91.1g

NOTES: Feel free to add grilled chicken, chickpeas, or your protein of choice to make it a complete meal.

2.2 Pomegranate and Walnut Arugula Salad

Preparation time	Cooking time	Servings
15 minutes	-	2

INGREDIENTS:

For Salad:

- 4 cups (120g) arugula
- 1 cup (160g) pomegranate seeds
- 1/2 cup (60g) walnuts, chopped
- 1/2 cup (60g) feta cheese, crumbled
- 1/2 cup (60g) red onion, thinly sliced

For Balsamic Vinaigrette (whisk or mix them well to ensure thorough blending):

- 4 tablespoons (60ml) extra virgin olive oil
- 2 tablespoons (30ml) balsamic vinegar
- 2 teaspoons honey
- 1 teaspoon Dijon mustard
- Salt and pepper to taste

INSTRUCTIONS:

For Pomegranate and Walnut Arugula Salad:

1. In a large bowl, place the arugula.
2. Sprinkle pomegranate seeds over the arugula.
3. Add chopped walnuts to the salad.
4. Sprinkle crumbled feta cheese over the salad.
5. Toss in thinly sliced red onion in the bowl.

For Balsamic Vinaigrette:

1. Toss the extra virgin olive oil, honey, Dijon mustard, balsamic vinegar, salt, and pepper in a small bowl. Blend until thoroughly blended.
2. After tasting the vinaigrette, taste and adjust the seasoning (salt, pepper, etc.) to your preference.
3. Drizzle the balsamic vinaigrette over the salad.
4. Toss the salad gently so all ingredients are coated with the vinaigrette.
5. Serve the Pomegranate and Walnut Arugula Salad immediately to enjoy its freshness.

Nutritional Information (per serving):

Calories: 2402 | Fat: 211.7g | Saturated Fat: 32g | Cholesterol: 22mg | Sodium: 933mg | Carbohydrate: 140.1g | Fiber: 20.9g | Protein: 23.3g

NOTES: Add grilled chicken or avocado slices for protein and creaminess.

2.3 Citrus Bliss Salad with Mixed Greens and Oranges

Preparation time	Cooking time	Servings
15 minutes	-	2

INGREDIENTS:

For Salad:

- 4 cups (120g) mixed salad greens (such as spinach, arugula, and romaine)
- 2 oranges, peeled and segmented
- 1/2 cup (60g) red onion, thinly sliced
- 1/2 cup (60g) feta cheese, crumbled
- 4 tablespoons (30g) sliced almonds, toasted

For Citrus Vinaigrette:

- 4 tablespoons (60ml) extra virgin olive oil
- 2 tablespoons (30ml) orange juice
- 2 tablespoons (30ml) lemon juice
- 2 teaspoons honey
- 1 teaspoon Dijon mustard
- Salt and pepper to taste

INSTRUCTIONS:

For Citrus Bliss Salad:

1. Combine the mixed salad greens in a large bowl.
2. Gently fold in the orange segments to the salad greens.
3. Add a red onion, cut thinly, to the salad.
4. Sprinkle crumbled feta cheese over the salad.
5. Scatter toasted sliced almonds on top for added crunch.

For Citrus Vinaigrette:

1. Whisk or mix the extra virgin olive oil, lemon and orange juices, honey, Dijon mustard, salt, and pepper well in a small bowl. Mix until well combined.
2. After tasting the vinaigrette, adjust the seasoning by adding additional honey, salt, or pepper to taste.
3. Drizzle the citrus vinaigrette over the salad just before serving.
4. Toss the salad carefully to coat it evenly with dressing.
5. Serve the Citrus Bliss Salad immediately to maintain the freshness and crunch.

Nutritional Information (per serving):

Calories: 3446 | Fat: 296.9g | Saturated Fat: 39.5g | Cholesterol: 22mg | Sodium: 948mg | Carbohydrate: 194.4g | Fiber: 43.6g | Protein: 59g

NOTES:

___
___
___
___

2.4 Mediterranean Greek Salad with Feta and Kalamata Olives

Preparation time	Cooking time	Servings
15 minutes	-	2

INGREDIENTS:

For Salad:

- 4 cups (120g) mixed salad greens
- 1 cup (150g) cherry tomatoes, halved
- 1/2 cup (60g) cucumber, diced
- 1/2 cup (60g) red bell pepper, diced
- 1/2 cup (60g) red onion, thinly sliced
- 4 ounces (120g) feta cheese, crumbled
- 1/2 cup (60g) Kalamata olives, pitted and halved
- Fresh oregano leaves, for garnish

For Greek Salad Dressing:

- 4 tablespoons (60ml) extra virgin olive oil
- 2 tablespoons (30ml) red wine vinegar
- 2 teaspoons dried oregano
- 2 cloves garlic, minced
- Salt and black pepper, to taste

INSTRUCTIONS:

For Greek Salad Dressing:

Combine the dried oregano, minced garlic, extra virgin olive oil, red wine vinegar, salt, and black pepper in a small bowl. Set aside.

Assemble Mediterranean Greek Salad:

1. Arrange the mixed salad greens onto a platter for presentation.
2. Scatter halved cherry tomatoes over the salad greens.
3. Add diced cucumber and red bell pepper to the salad.
4. Sprinkle thinly sliced red onion over the salad.
5. Crumble feta cheese over the salad.
6. Distribute halved Kalamata olives across the salad.
7. Over the salad, drizzle the Greek Salad Dressing.
8. Add some fresh oregano leaves as a garnish for an additional flavor boost.
9. Make sure the salad is evenly covered with the dressing by gently tossing it.

Nutritional Information (per serving):

Calories: 2825 | Fat: 244.7g | Saturated Fat: 60.2g | Cholesterol: 178mg | Sodium: 2566mg | Carbohydrate: 154.5g | Fiber: 60.6g | Protein: 55.2g

NOTES: If you would like more protein, feel free to add grilled chicken or shrimp.

2.5 Grilled Chicken Caesar Salad with Whole-grain Croutons

Preparation time	Cooking time	Servings
20 minutes	10 minutes	2

INGREDIENTS:

For Salad:

- 2 boneless, skinless chicken breasts
- Salt and black pepper, to taste
- 2 tablespoons (30ml) olive oil
- 2 heads romaine lettuce, washed and chopped
- 1/2 cup (60g) cherry tomatoes, halved
- 1/2 cup (60g) Parmesan cheese, shaved

For Whole-grain Croutons:

- 2 cups (80g) whole-grain bread, cut into cubes
- 2 tablespoons (30ml) olive oil
- 1 teaspoon garlic powder
- 1 teaspoon dried oregano
- Salt and black pepper, to taste

For Caesar Dressing:

- 4 tablespoons (60ml) mayonnaise
- 2 tablespoons (30ml) Dijon mustard
- 2 cloves garlic, minced
- 2 tablespoons (30ml) lemon juice
- 1/2 cup (120ml) extra virgin olive oil
- Salt and black pepper, to taste

INSTRUCTIONS:

For Grilled Chicken:

1. Add some black pepper and salt to the chicken breast to season it.
2. Heat olive oil over medium-high heat in a grill pan or outdoor grill. The chicken breast should be cooked through after 6 to 8 minutes on each side of the grill. Allow it to rest for a few minutes before slicing.

For Whole-grain Croutons:

1. Preheat the oven to 375°F (190°C).
2. Toss the whole-grain bread cubes with olive oil, garlic powder, dried oregano, salt, and black pepper in a bowl.
3. Line a baking sheet with the seasoned bread cubes, and bake for 10 to 12 minutes until golden brown and crisp. Allow them to cool.

For Caesar Dressing:

Whisk or blend the mayonnaise, Dijon mustard, minced garlic, lemon juice, and extra virgin olive oil thoroughly in a small bowl for a smooth dressing. Season with salt and black pepper to taste.

Assemble Grilled Chicken Caesar Salad:

1. Chop the washed and dried romaine lettuce and place it in a large bowl.
2. Add halved cherry tomatoes to the bowl.
3. Shave Parmesan cheese over the salad using a vegetable peeler.
4. After grilling, cut the chicken breast into slices and arrange it over the salad.

5. Sprinkle the whole-grain croutons over the salad.
6. Drizzle the Caesar dressing over the salad.
7. Make sure the salad is evenly covered with the dressing by gently tossing it.

Nutritional Information (per serving):

Calories: 3409 | Fat: 237.4g | Saturated Fat: 39.7g | Cholesterol: 159mg | Sodium: 3547mg | Carbohydrate: 279.6g | Fiber: 68.6g | Protein: 91.8g

NOTES: Customize the salad by adding anchovies or extra vegetables per your preferences.

_____
_____
_____
_____

2.6 Watermelon and Feta Salad with Mint

Preparation time	Cooking time	Servings
10 minutes	-	2

INGREDIENTS:

- 4 cups (600g) watermelon, cubed
- 4 ounces (120g) feta cheese, crumbled
- Fresh mint leaves, torn or chopped, to taste
- 2 tablespoons (30ml) extra virgin olive oil
- 2 tablespoons (30ml) balsamic glaze
- Salt and black pepper, to taste

INSTRUCTIONS:

1. Cube the watermelon into bite-sized pieces.
2. Crumble the feta cheese.
3. The watermelon cubes should be put on a serving platter.
4. Sprinkle crumbled feta cheese over the watermelon.
5. Toss torn or chopped fresh mint leaves over the salad.
6. Pour balsamic glaze and extra virgin olive oil over the salad.
7. Season with salt and black pepper to taste.
8. Toss the salad gently to include all the ingredients.

Nutritional Information (per serving):

Calories: 1538 | Fat: 138.2g | Saturated Fat: 43.9g | Cholesterol: 178mg | Sodium: 2272mg | Carbohydrate: 59.8g | Fiber: 17.4g | Protein: 36.7g

NOTES: Adjust the amount of mint, olive oil, and balsamic glaze according to your taste preferences.

_____
_____
_____
_____

2.7 Roasted Beet and Goat Cheese Salad with Balsamic Glaze

Preparation time	Cooking time	Servings
15 minutes	45 minutes (including roasting time for beets)	2

INGREDIENTS:

For Roasted Beets:

- 4 medium-sized beets, peeled and cubed
- 2 tablespoons (30ml) olive oil
- Salt and black pepper, to taste

For Salad:

- 4 cups (120g) mixed salad greens
- 4 ounces (120g) goat cheese, crumbled
- 4 tablespoons (60g) walnuts, chopped
- Fresh mint leaves, for garnish (optional)

For Balsamic Glaze:

- 1/2 cup (120ml) balsamic vinegar
- 2 tablespoons (30ml) honey

INSTRUCTIONS:

For Roasted Beets:

1. Preheat the oven to 400°F (200°C).
2. Peel and cube the beets.
3. Toss the beet cubes with olive oil, salt, and black pepper. After putting the beets on a baking sheet, roast them in a preheated oven for 25 to 30 minutes or until they are soft and starting to caramelize. Allow them to cool.

For Balsamic Glaze:

Honey and balsamic vinegar should be combined in a small pot. Stirring occasionally, bring the mixture to a simmer over medium heat. Simmer for 8-10 minutes or until the glaze thickens. Remove from heat and let it cool.

Note: The glaze will continue to thicken as it cools, so you should remove it from the heat when it reaches its desired consistency

Assemble Roasted Beet and Goat Cheese Salad:

1. Arrange the mixed salad greens onto a platter for presentation.
2. Scatter the roasted beet cubes over the salad greens.
3. Crumble goat cheese over the salad.
4. Sprinkle chopped walnuts on top.
5. Drizzle the balsamic glaze over the salad.
6. Garnish with fresh mint leaves if desired.

Nutritional Information (per serving):

Calories: 3519 | Fat: 285g | Saturated Fat: 70g | Cholesterol: 210mg |
Sodium: 944mg | Carbohydrate: 169.8g | Fiber: 34.5g | Protein: 122.5g

NOTES:
- Customize the salad by adding arugula or spinach for extra greens.
- Consider adding a sprinkle of black sesame seeds for an additional touch.

2.8 Caprese Salad with Heirloom Tomatoes and Basil

Preparation time	Cooking time	Servings
10 minutes	-	2

INGREDIENTS:
- 2 cups (400g) heirloom tomatoes, sliced
- 1 cup (240g) fresh mozzarella cheese, sliced
- Fresh basil leaves
- 4 tablespoons (60ml) extra virgin olive oil
- 2 tablespoons (30ml) balsamic glaze
- Salt and pepper to taste

INSTRUCTIONS:
1. Wash and slice the heirloom tomatoes into rounds.
2. Slice the fresh mozzarella cheese into rounds of similar thickness to the tomatoes.
3. Arrange the heirloom tomato and fresh mozzarella slices on a serving plate, alternating them for a visually appealing presentation.
4. Place a few fresh basil leaves in between the mozzarella and tomato slices.
5. Olive oil extra virgin should be drizzled over the salad.
6. Drizzle balsamic glaze over the tomato and mozzarella slices.
7. Sprinkle salt and pepper to taste.

Nutritional Information (per serving):

Calories: 1958 | Fat: 202.1g | Saturated Fat: 31.7g | Cholesterol: 22mg |
Sodium: 363mg | Carbohydrate: 68.9g | Fiber: 28.4g | Protein: 16.1g

NOTES:
- Use a high-quality balsamic glaze for the best flavor.
- Add a dash of freshly ground black pepper or a sprinkle of dried oregano for extra seasoning.

2.9 Spinach and Strawberry Salad with Poppy Seed Dressing

Preparation time	Cooking time	Servings
15 minutes	-	2

INGREDIENTS:

For Salad:

- 4 cups (120g) fresh spinach leaves, washed and dried
- 2 cups (300g) strawberries, hulled and sliced
- 1/2 cup (60g) red onion, thinly sliced
- 1/2 cup (60g) feta cheese, crumbled
- 4 tablespoons (60g) sliced almonds, toasted

For Poppy Seed Dressing:

- 4 tablespoons (60ml) olive oil
- 2 tablespoons (30ml) balsamic vinegar
- 2 tablespoons (30ml) honey
- 2 teaspoons poppy seeds
- Salt and black pepper, to taste

INSTRUCTIONS:

For Poppy Seed Dressing:

Mix the olive oil, balsamic vinegar, honey, poppy seeds, salt, and black pepper in a small bowl. Set aside.

Assemble Spinach and Strawberry Salad:

1. Place the fresh spinach leaves on a serving plate.
2. Scatter sliced strawberries over the spinach.
3. Sprinkle thinly sliced red onion over the salad.
4. Crumble feta cheese over the salad.
5. Sprinkle toasted sliced almonds over the salad for a crunchy texture.
6. Over the salad, drizzle the poppy seed dressing.
7. Make sure the salad is evenly covered with the dressing by gently tossing it.

Nutritional Information (per serving):

Calories: 3897 | Fat: 339.4g | Saturated Fat: 43.5g | Cholesterol: 22mg | Sodium: 493mg | Carbohydrate: 200.6g | Fiber: 55.4g | Protein: 76.3g

NOTES: To add more protein, add grilled chicken or shrimp.

CHAPTER 3: WHOLESOME SOUPS

These wholesome soups are crafted to comfort, nourish, and bring a symphony of flavors to your table. Enjoy the heartiness and warmth!

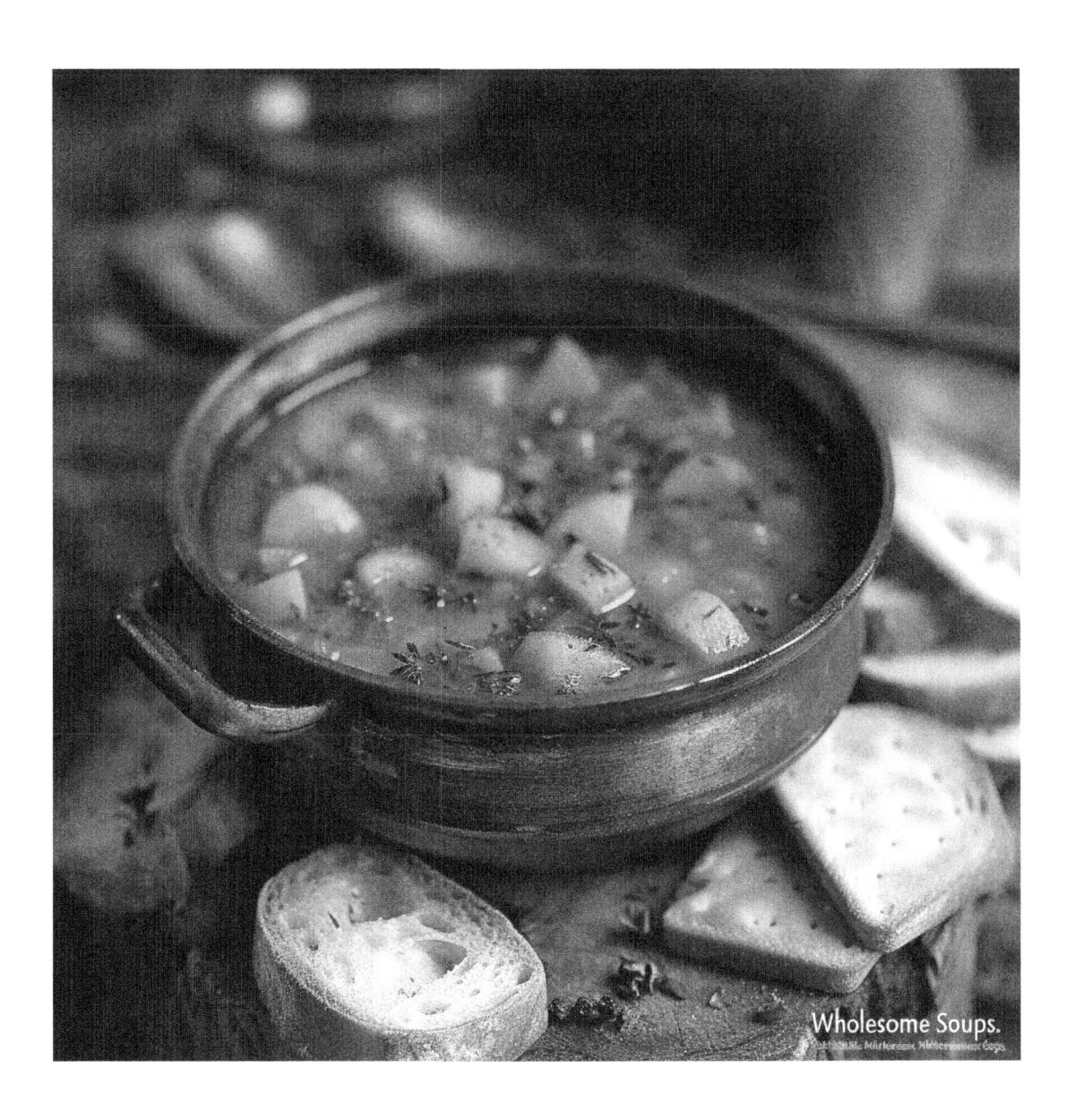

3.1 Moroccan Chickpea Stew with Cilantro Drizzle

Preparation time	Cooking time	Servings
20 minutes	30 minutes	2

INGREDIENTS:

For the Stew:

- 1 cup (180g) cooked chickpeas
- 1/2 cup (60g) carrot, diced
- 1/2 cup (60g) red bell pepper, diced
- 1/2 cup (60g) zucchini, diced
- 1/2 cup (60g) eggplant, diced
- 1/2 cup (60g) onion, finely chopped
- 2 cloves garlic, minced
- 2 tablespoons (30ml) olive oil
- 2 teaspoons ground cumin
- 1 teaspoon ground coriander
- 1 teaspoon paprika
- 1/2 teaspoon ground cinnamon
- 2 cups (480ml) vegetable broth
- Salt and black pepper, to taste
- Fresh cilantro for garnish

For the Cilantro Drizzle:

- 4 tablespoons (60g) fresh cilantro, chopped
- 2 tablespoons (30ml) olive oil
- 2 teaspoons lemon juice
- Salt, to taste

INSTRUCTIONS:

1. Dice the carrot, red bell pepper, zucchini, eggplant, and finely chop the onion.
2. In a saucepan of moderate size, warm the olive oil over medium heat. Add chopped onion and minced garlic, sautéing until fragrant.
3. Add diced carrot, red bell pepper, zucchini, and eggplant to the pot. The vegetables should start to soften after a few minutes of sautéing.
4. Sprinkle ground cumin, coriander, paprika, and cinnamon over the vegetables. Stir to coat evenly.
5. Add cooked chickpeas to the pot, mixing them with the vegetables and spices.
6. Pour vegetable broth into the pot, ensuring it covers the vegetables and chickpeas. Bring the mixture to a gentle boil.
7. Reduce heat to low, cover, and let the stew simmer for 15-20 minutes or until the vegetables are tender.
8. Season the stew with salt and black pepper to taste.
9. To make the cilantro drizzle, combine fresh cilantro, olive oil, lemon juice, and a little salt in a small bowl.
10. Drizzle the cilantro mixture over the stew and garnish with fresh cilantro leaves.

Nutritional Information (per serving):

Calories: 1944 | Fat: 129.4g | Saturated Fat: 17.9g | Cholesterol: 0mg | Sodium: 20025mg | Carbohydrate: 201.7g | Fiber: 72.3g | Protein: 54.2g

NOTES:

- Adapt the amount of spice to your taste.
- Serve the stew over couscous or quinoa for a complete meal.

3.2 Spinach and Orzo Lemon Drop Soup

Preparation time	Cooking time	Servings
15 minutes	20 minutes	2

INGREDIENTS:

- 1/2 cup (60g) orzo pasta
- 2 cups (60g) fresh spinach leaves
- 1/2 cup (60g) carrot, finely diced
- 1/2 cup (60g) celery, finely diced
- 1/2 cup (60g) onion, finely chopped
- 2 cloves garlic, minced
- 2 tablespoons (30ml) olive oil
- 8 cups (1920ml) vegetable broth
- Juice of 2 lemons
- Zest of 2 lemons
- 1/2 teaspoon dried thyme
- Salt and black pepper, to taste
- Fresh dill for garnish

INSTRUCTIONS:

1. Finely chop onion, garlic, carrot, and celery. Rinse fresh spinach leaves.
2. In a saucepan of moderate size, warm the olive oil over medium heat. Add chopped onion and minced garlic, sautéing until fragrant.
3. Add diced carrot, celery, and orzo pasta to the pot. The veggies should start to soften after a few minutes of sautéing.
4. Cover the orzo and veggies with vegetable broth after adding it to the saucepan. Bring the mixture to a gentle boil.
5. Reduce heat to low, cover, and let the soup simmer for 10-15 minutes or until the orzo is cooked.
6. Stir in fresh spinach leaves, allowing them to wilt into the soup.
7. Squeeze the juice of one lemon into the soup. Add lemon zest and dried thyme. Stir well.
8. Season the soup with salt and black pepper to taste.

Nutritional Information (per serving):

Calories: 1520 | Fat: 102.8g | Saturated Fat: 15.5g | Cholesterol: 18mg | Sodium: 1552mg | Carbohydrate: 149.7g | Fiber: 35.2g | Protein: 38.5g

NOTES:

- Adjust the lemon juice and zest according to your taste preferences.
- Feel free to add a tiny pinch of red pepper flakes for extra spiciness.

3.3 Tomato Basil Harmony Soup with Whole Wheat Croutons

Preparation time	Cooking time	Servings
15 minutes	30 minutes	2

INGREDIENTS:

For Tomato Basil Soup:

- 2 tablespoons (30ml) olive oil
- 1/2 cup (60g) onion, finely chopped
- 2 cloves garlic, minced
- 1/2 teaspoon dried oregano
- 1/2 teaspoon dried basil
- 1/2 teaspoon dried thyme
- 1/2 teaspoon smoked paprika
- 1/2 teaspoon of optionally hot red pepper flakes
- 2 cans (14 oz / 400g each) diced tomatoes, undrained
- 2 cups (480ml) vegetable broth
- Salt and black pepper, to taste
- Fresh basil leaves for garnish

For Whole Wheat Croutons:

- 2 slices whole wheat bread, cubed
- 2 teaspoons olive oil
- 1/2 teaspoon garlic powder
- 1/2 teaspoon dried oregano
- Pinch of salt

INSTRUCTIONS:

For Tomato Basil Soup:

1. Olive oil should be heated to a medium temperature in a medium pot. Add chopped onion and garlic, sautéing until fragrant and translucent.
2. Add the smoked paprika, red pepper flakes, dried oregano, dried basil, and dried thyme (if using). Saute for one more minute.
3. Add the diced tomatoes, juice, and vegetable broth from the can. Raise the mixture to a simmer.
4. Turn down the heat to low, cover, and simmer the soup for 15 to 20 minutes to let the flavors combine.
5. Season the soup with salt and black pepper to taste.
6. While the soup is simmering, prepare the whole wheat croutons.

For Whole Wheat Croutons:

1. Cut the whole wheat bread into cubes.
2. Combine the bread cubes, dried oregano, olive oil, and a small amount of salt in a bowl.
3. Heat a skillet over medium heat. Toast the seasoned bread cubes until they become golden brown and crisp.

Assemble and Serve:

1. Ladle the Tomato Basil Harmony Soup into a bowl.
2. Garnish the soup with whole wheat croutons.
3. Finish by garnishing the soup with fresh basil leaves.

Nutritional Information (per serving):

Calories: 1894 | Fat: 124.4g | Saturated Fat: 19.2g | Cholesterol: 0mg |

Sodium: 20802mg | Carbohydrate: 197.1g | Fiber: 62.9g | Protein: 44.7g

NOTES:
- If necessary, add additional stock to the soup to change its consistency.
- Feel free to customize the croutons with your favorite herbs and spices.

___

3.4 Minestrone Medley Soup with Garden Vegetables

Preparation time	Cooking time	Servings
20 minutes	25 minutes	2

INGREDIENTS:

- 2 tablespoons (30ml) olive oil
- 1/2 cup (60g) onion, finely chopped
- 2 cloves garlic, minced
- 1/2 cup (60g) carrot, diced
- 1/2 cup (60g) celery, diced
- 1/2 cup (60g) zucchini, diced
- 1/2 cup (60g) canned cannellini beans, drained and rinsed
- 1/2 cup (60g) canned diced tomatoes
- 1 teaspoon dried oregano
- 1 teaspoon dried basil
- 1/2 teaspoon dried thyme
- Salt and black pepper, to taste
- 2 cups (480ml) vegetable broth
- 1/2 cup (60g) small pasta (e.g., ditalini or small shells)
- 1/2 cup (60g) fresh spinach, chopped
- Grated Parmesan cheese, for garnish (optional)

INSTRUCTIONS:

1. Olive oil should be heated to a medium temperature in a medium-sized pot. Add chopped onion and garlic, sautéing until fragrant and translucent.
2. Stir in diced carrot, celery, zucchini, cannellini beans, and canned tomatoes.
3. Add dried oregano, basil, dried thyme, salt, and black pepper. Stir to combine.
4. Pour vegetable broth into the pot, bringing the mixture to a gentle boil.
5. Stir in the small pasta of your choice. Cook according to package instructions or until pasta is al dente.
6. Add chopped fresh spinach to the soup, letting it wilt into the mixture.
7. After tasting the soup, add more salt or pepper, if preferred, to the seasoning.
8. Ladle the Minestrone Medley Soup into a bowl. Optionally, garnish with grated Parmesan cheese.

Nutritional Information (per serving):

Calories: 1536 | Fat: 104.1g | Saturated Fat: 16.2g | Cholesterol: 0mg | Sodium: 448mg | Carbohydrate: 157.2g | Fiber: 56.6g | Protein: 34.3g

NOTES: For an additional taste boost, consider including a small amount of balsamic vinegar.

3.5 Creamy Cauliflower and Leek Soup

Preparation time	Cooking time	Servings
15 minutes	30 minutes	2

INGREDIENTS:

- 2 cups (300g) cauliflower florets
- 1/2 cup (60g) leek, thinly sliced
- 2 cloves garlic, minced
- 2 tablespoons (30ml) olive oil
- 1/2 teaspoon dried thyme
- 1/2 teaspoon dried rosemary
- 1/2 teaspoon ground nutmeg
- 4 cups (960ml) vegetable broth
- 1 cup (240ml) unsweetened almond milk
- Salt and black pepper, to taste
- Fresh chives, for garnish

INSTRUCTIONS:

1. Slice the leek very thinly and chop the cauliflower into tiny florets.
2. In a medium pot set over medium heat, warm the olive oil. Add minced garlic and sliced leek, sautéing until the leek becomes tender.
3. Add cauliflower florets to the pot. Sauté for a few minutes until the cauliflower starts to brown slightly.
4. Sprinkle dried thyme, dried rosemary, and ground nutmeg over the vegetables. Stir to coat evenly.
5. Cover the vegetables in the pot with vegetable broth. Bring the mixture to a gentle boil.
6. After turning down the heat to low and covering, simmer the soup for 15 to 20 minutes or until the cauliflower is tender.
7. Blend the soup until it's smooth and creamy, either with an immersion blender or by moving it to a countertop blender.
8. Stir in unsweetened almond milk to achieve the desired creamy consistency.
9. Season the soup with salt and black pepper to taste.
10. Garnish with Fresh Chives:
11. Garnish with fresh chives for a burst of oniony freshness.

Nutritional Information (per serving):

Calories: 1455 | Fat: 112.6g | Saturated Fat: 23.4g | Cholesterol: 0mg | Sodium: 778mg | Carbohydrate: 122g | Fiber: 44.9g | Protein: 25g

NOTES:_____
_____
_____
_____

3.6 Spicy Black Bean and Sweet Potato Soup

Preparation time	Cooking time	Servings
15 minutes	30 minutes	2

INGREDIENTS:

- 1 cup (200g) black beans, cooked
- 1 cup (150g) sweet potato, diced
- 1/2 cup (60g) red bell pepper, diced
- 1/2 cup (60g) corn kernels (fresh or frozen)
- 1/2 cup (60g) onion, finely chopped
- 2 cloves garlic, minced
- 2 tablespoons (30ml) olive oil
- 2 teaspoons ground cumin
- 1 teaspoon chili powder
- 1/2 teaspoon smoked paprika
- 4 cups (960ml) vegetable broth
- Salt and black pepper, to taste
- Fresh cilantro for garnish
- Avocado slices for topping (optional)

INSTRUCTIONS:

1. Dice sweet potato, red bell pepper, and onion. Rinse and drain the cooked black beans.
2. In a saucepan of moderate size, warm the olive oil over medium heat. Add chopped onion and minced garlic, sautéing until fragrant.
3. Add diced sweet potato, red bell pepper, and corn kernels to the pot. The veggies should start to soften after a few minutes of sautéing.
4. Sprinkle ground cumin, chili powder, and smoked paprika over the vegetables. Stir to coat evenly.
5. Add cooked black beans to the pot, mixing them with the vegetables and spices.
6. Cover the veggies and beans in the saucepan with vegetable broth. Bring the mixture to a gentle boil.
7. Reduce heat to low, cover, and let the soup simmer for 15-20 minutes or until the sweet potatoes are tender.
8. Season the soup with salt and black pepper to taste.
9. For a taste explosion of herbaceous flavor, garnish with fresh cilantro leaves.
10. Top with Avocado (Optional): For added creaminess, top the soup with sliced avocado if desired.

Nutritional Information (per serving):

Calories: 2094 | Fat: 141.9g | Saturated Fat: 20.1g | Cholesterol: 0mg | Sodium: 1410mg | Carbohydrate: 211.3g | Fiber: 68.3g | Protein: 59.2g

NOTES:_____
_____
_____
_____

3.7 Chicken and Vegetable Broth Elixir

Preparation time	Cooking time	Servings
10 minutes	1 hour 30 minutes	2

INGREDIENTS:

- 2 cups (480ml) low-sodium chicken broth
- 1/2 cup (60g) cooked chicken breast, shredded
- 1/2 cup (60g) carrot, thinly sliced
- 1/2 cup (60g) celery, thinly sliced
- 1/2 cup (60g) onion, finely chopped
- 2 cloves garlic, minced
- 1/2 teaspoon ground turmeric
- 1/2 teaspoon ground ginger
- 1/2 teaspoon dried rosemary
- 1/2 teaspoon dried thyme
- Salt and black pepper, to taste
- Fresh parsley for garnish

INSTRUCTIONS:

1. Shred the cooked chicken breast and thinly slice the carrot and celery.
2. Add a splash of water or a small amount of olive oil in a medium sized-pot. Sauté chopped onion and minced garlic until fragrant.
3. Add sliced carrots and celery to the pot. Sauté for a few minutes until they start to soften.
4. Pour low-sodium chicken broth into the pot, bringing it to a gentle simmer.
5. Stir in shredded cooked chicken breast.
6. Sprinkle ground turmeric, ginger, rosemary, dried thyme, salt, and black pepper into the broth. Stir to combine.
7. Let the elixir simmer for 10-15 minutes to allow the flavors to meld.
8. After tasting the soup, taste again and adjust the seasoning by adding additional salt or pepper to taste.
9. For a burst of herbaceous taste, garnish with fresh parsley.

Nutritional Information (per serving):

Calories: 681 | Fat: 12.9g | Saturated Fat: 4.5g | Cholesterol: 16mg | Sodium: 191mg | Carbohydrate: 140.5g | Fiber: 46.9g | Protein: 27.9g

NOTES:

- For added nutritional content, try other vegetables like spinach or kale.
- Consider a squeeze of lemon for a touch of acidity.

_____
_____
_____
_____

3.8 Lentil and Spinach Delight Soup

Preparation time	Cooking time	Servings
15 minutes	40 minutes	2

INGREDIENTS:

- 1/2 cup (100g) dried green or brown lentils, rinsed
- 2 tablespoons (30ml) olive oil
- 1/2 cup (60g) onion, finely chopped
- 2 cloves garlic, minced
- 1/2 cup (60g) carrot, diced
- 1/2 cup (60g) celery, diced
- 1/2 teaspoon ground cumin
- 1/2 teaspoon ground coriander
- 1/2 teaspoon smoked paprika
- 1/2 teaspoon dried thyme
- Salt and black pepper, to taste
- 4 cups (960ml) vegetable broth
- 1 cup (120g) fresh spinach leaves, chopped
- 2 tablespoons (30ml) lemon juice (optional)

INSTRUCTIONS:

1. Rinse dried lentils under cold water.
2. In a medium-sized pot, warm the olive oil. Add chopped onion and garlic, sautéing until fragrant and translucent.
3. Stir in diced carrot, celery, cumin, ground coriander, smoked paprika, dried thyme, salt, and black pepper.
4. Add rinsed lentils to the pot and stir to combine with the vegetables and spices.
5. Pour vegetable broth into the pot, bringing the mixture to a gentle boil.
6. Reduce heat to low, cover, and let the soup simmer for about 20-25 minutes or until lentils are tender.
7. Stir in chopped fresh spinach and let it wilt into the soup.
8. After tasting the soup, adjust the seasoning. Add more salt or pepper if desired.
9. If desired, squeeze lemon juice into the soup for a refreshing kick.

Nutritional Information (per serving):

Calories: 1484 | Fat: 108.7g | Saturated Fat: 16.7g | Cholesterol: 0mg | Sodium: 848mg | Carbohydrate: 129.9g | Fiber: 42.6g | Protein: 35.2g

NOTES:

- To personalize the soup, feel free to add more veggies, such as tomatoes or bell peppers.
- For added richness, consider finishing with a drizzle of extra virgin olive oil.

3.9 Butternut Squash and Apple Bisque

Preparation time	Cooking time	Servings
20 minutes	30 minutes (including roasting time for butternut squash)	2

INGREDIENTS:

- 2 cups (300g) butternut squash, peeled and diced
- 1 cup (150g) apple, peeled and diced
- 1/2 cup (60g) onion, finely chopped
- 2 tablespoons (30ml) olive oil
- 1/2 teaspoon ground cinnamon
- 1/2 teaspoon ground nutmeg
- 1/2 teaspoon dried sage
- 1/2 teaspoon dried thyme
- 2 cups (480ml) vegetable broth
- 1 cup (240ml) unsweetened almond milk
- Salt and black pepper, to taste
- 2 tablespoons (30ml) maple syrup (optional for sweetness)
- Chopped fresh parsley for garnish

INSTRUCTIONS:

1. Dice and peel the apple and butternut squash.
2. Olive oil should be heated to a medium temperature in a medium-sized pot. Add chopped onion and sauté until translucent.
3. Add diced butternut squash and apple to the pot. Sauté for 5 minutes, allowing them to caramelize slightly.
4. Sprinkle ground cinnamon, ground nutmeg, dried sage, and dried thyme over the vegetables. Stir to coat evenly.
5. Pour vegetable broth into the pot, ensuring it covers the vegetables. Bring the mixture to a gentle boil.
6. After lowering the heat to low and covering the mixture, simmer the ingredients for 15 to 20 minutes or until the butternut squash is soft.
7. Blend the mixture until it's smooth and creamy, either with an immersion blender or by moving it to a tabletop blender.
8. Stir in unsweetened almond milk to achieve the desired consistency.
9. Season the bisque with salt and black pepper to taste. Add maple syrup if a touch of sweetness is desired.

Nutritional Information (per serving):

Calories: 1684 | Fat: 111.6g | Saturated Fat: 23.2g | Cholesterol: 0mg | Sodium: 442mg | Carbohydrate: 196.5g | Fiber: 58.2g | Protein: 18.2g

NOTES: Adjust the sweetness and consistency according to your taste preferences.

_____
_____
_____
_____

CHAPTER 4: LEAN PROTEINS

These nutrient-dense, tasty lean protein dishes provide a range of choices for anybody trying to include more healthful protein sources. Enjoy the balance of flavors and textures!

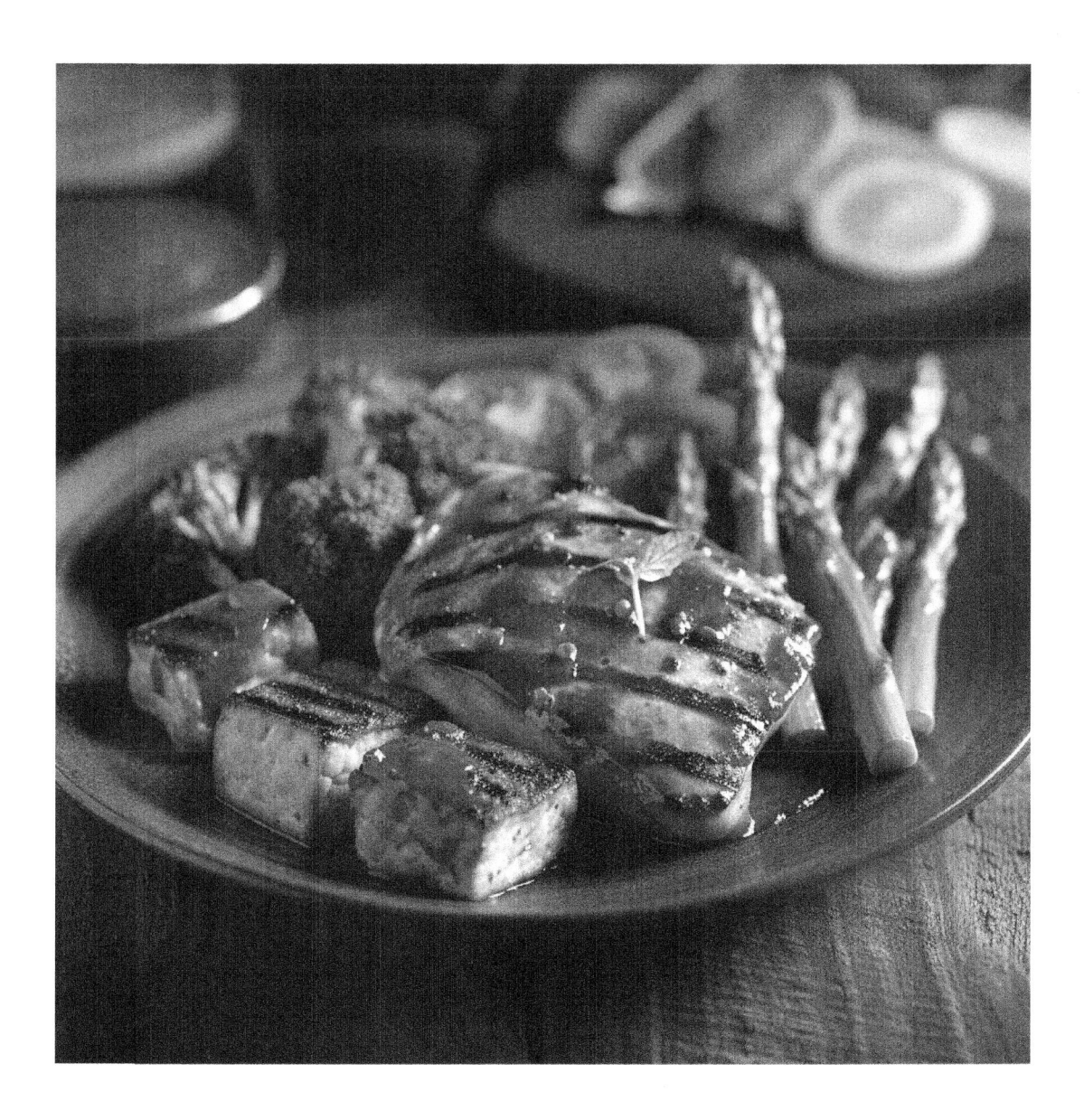

4.1 Grilled Lemon Herb Salmon

Preparation time	Cooking time	Servings
10 minutes	15 minutes	2

INGREDIENTS:

- 2 salmon fillets (about 12 oz or 340g total)
- 2 tablespoons (30ml) olive oil
- 2 tablespoons (30ml) lemon juice
- 2 cloves garlic, minced
- 1 teaspoon dried dill
- 1 teaspoon dried parsley
- Salt and black pepper, to taste
- Lemon slices, for garnish
- Fresh parsley, chopped, for garnish

INSTRUCTIONS:

1. Utilizing paper towels, pat dry the salmon fillet. Transfer it to a shallow dish or platter.
2. Olive oil, lemon juice, minced garlic, dried dill, dried parsley, salt, and black pepper should all be combined in a small dish to form the marinade.
3. Marinade the flavors for at least 15 to 30 minutes to allow them to seep in.
4. Preheat your grill to medium-high heat.
5. Place the marinated salmon fillet on the preheated grill. Grill the salmon for 3–4 minutes on each side or until it reaches the doneness you like.
6. For extra flavor, baste the salmon with the leftover marinade while cooking.
7. When a fork readily flakes into the salmon, it's done. Be cautious not to overcook it to keep it moist and tender.
8. Transfer the grilled lemon herb salmon to a plate. Add lemon slices and finely chopped fresh parsley as garnish.

Nutritional Information (per serving):

Calories: 1414 | Fat: 105.2g | Saturated Fat: 15.8g | Cholesterol: 44mg | Sodium: 263mg | Carbohydrate: 104.7g | Fiber: 28.4g | Protein: 45.7g

NOTES:

- Experiment with additional herbs like thyme or rosemary for extra aroma.
- Serve with roasted vegetables or a light salad for a complete meal.

_____
_____
_____
_____

4.2 Turkey and Quinoa Stuffed Bell Peppers

Preparation time	Cooking time	Servings
20 minutes	40 minutes	2

INGREDIENTS:

- 2 large bell peppers (any color)
- 1 cup (180g) lean ground turkey
- 1/2 cup (100g) quinoa, cooked
- 1/2 cup (60g) onion, finely chopped
- 1/2 cup (60g) tomato, diced
- 2 cloves garlic, minced
- 1/2 teaspoon ground cumin
- 1/2 teaspoon paprika
- Salt and black pepper, to taste
- 1/2 cup (60g) shredded mozzarella cheese
- Fresh parsley, chopped, for garnish

INSTRUCTIONS:

1. Preheat your oven to 375°F (190°C).
2. Cut the top off the bell pepper and remove seeds and membranes. Lightly season the inside with a pinch of salt.
3. In a skillet over medium heat, sauté chopped onion and minced garlic until softened.
4. Cook the ground turkey in the skillet until it becomes golden. Season with ground cumin, paprika, salt, and black pepper.
5. Stir in cooked quinoa and diced tomato. Cook for an additional 2-3 minutes until well combined.
6. Stuff the hollowed bell pepper with the turkey and quinoa mixture.
7. Top the filled bell pepper with shredded mozzarella cheese.
8. Once soft, stir the bell pepper into a baking dish and bake it in a preheated oven for 20 to 25 minutes.
9. The cheese should be melted, and the pepper should be soft but still have some structure when the filled bell pepper is done.

Nutritional Information (per serving):

Calories: 696 | Fat: 18.1g | Saturated Fat: 3.6g | Cholesterol: 39mg | Sodium: 205mg | Carbohydrate: 122.2g | Fiber: 33.2g | Protein: 38.5g

NOTES:

- Customize the seasoning, adding herbs like oregano or thyme for extra flavor.
- Pair with a side of mixed greens or a light salad for a balanced meal.

4.3 Baked Chicken Breast with Herbed Yogurt Marinade

Preparation time	Cooking time	Servings
15 minutes	30 minutes	2

INGREDIENTS:

- 2 boneless, skinless chicken breasts (about 12 oz or 340g total)
- 1/2 cup (120g) Greek yogurt
- 2 tablespoons (30ml) olive oil
- 2 cloves garlic, minced
- 2 teaspoons dried oregano
- 2 teaspoons dried thyme
- 1 teaspoon dried rosemary
- 1 teaspoon paprika
- Salt and black pepper, to taste
- Lemon wedges for serving
- Fresh parsley, chopped, for garnish

INSTRUCTIONS:

1. Preheat your oven to 400°F (200°C).
2. Using paper towels, pat dry the chicken breast. Place it in a shallow dish or a resealable plastic bag.
3. To make the marinade, combine Greek yogurt, olive oil, minced garlic, dried thyme, dried rosemary, paprika, salt, and black pepper in a dish.
4. Spread the yogurt marinade over the chicken breast, ensuring it's well-coated. Let it marinate for at least 30 minutes to allow the flavors to infuse.
5. Arrange the marinated chicken breast onto a parchment paper-lined baking sheet. After baking the chicken for 20 to 25 minutes in a preheated oven, its internal temperature should reach 165°F (74°C).
6. The chicken is done when it's no longer pink in the center, and the juices run clear.
7. Let the baked chicken breast rest for a few minutes before slicing. Garnish with fresh chopped parsley.
8. For an added zesty taste, serve the roasted chicken breast with lemon wedges.

Nutritional Information (per serving):

Calories: 3032 | Fat: 171.1g | Saturated Fat: 36.3g | Cholesterol: 535mg | Sodium: 20061mg | Carbohydrate: 230.2g | Fiber: 125g | Protein: 214.4g

NOTES:

- If you want a little heat, add a pinch of red pepper flakes.
- Adjust the spices and herbs to your personal preference.

_____
_____
_____
_____

4.4 Seared Tuna Steaks with Sesame Soy Glaze

Preparation time	Cooking time	Servings
15 minutes	15 minutes	2

INGREDIENTS:

- 2 tuna steaks (about 12 oz or 340g total)
- 2 tablespoons (30ml) soy sauce
- 2 tablespoons (30ml) sesame oil
- 2 tablespoons (30ml) rice vinegar
- 2 teaspoons honey
- 2 cloves garlic, minced
- 2 teaspoons fresh ginger, grated
- 2 tablespoons sesame seeds
- Green onions, sliced, for garnish
- Sesame seeds, for garnish

INSTRUCTIONS:

1. Using paper towels, pat dry the tuna steak. Ensure it's at room temperature for even cooking.
2. Whisk together soy sauce, sesame oil, rice vinegar, honey, minced garlic, and grated ginger in a small bowl to create the glaze.
3. Transfer half of the sesame soy glaze onto a shallow plate and cover the tuna steak. Let it marinate for about 15-30 minutes.
4. A skillet or nonstick pan should be heated to medium-high heat.
5. Remove the tuna from the marinade and sprinkle sesame seeds on both sides. Sear the tuna steak for 1-2 minutes on each side for medium-rare, and adjust the cooking time to your liking.
6. Brush the remaining sesame soy glaze over the tuna during the last minute of cooking.
7. The tuna is done when the edges are seared, and the center remains pink and slightly translucent.
8. Allow the seared tuna to rest for a few minutes before slicing. Garnish with sliced green onions and additional sesame seeds.

Nutritional Information (per serving):

Calories: 3501 | Fat: 193.9g | Saturated Fat: 32.9g | Cholesterol: 294mg | Sodium: 6009mg | Carbohydrate: 221g | Fiber: 28.7g | Protein: 220.2g

NOTES:

- Adjust the honey and soy sauce levels based on your desired sweetness and saltiness.
- For a full dinner, serve over sautéed vegetables or steaming rice.

4.5 Citrus-Marinated Grilled Shrimp Skewers

Preparation time	Cooking time	Servings
15 minutes	10 minutes	2

INGREDIENTS:

- 12-16 large shrimp, peeled and deveined
- 2 tablespoons (30ml) olive oil
- Zest and juice of 2 lemons
- Zest and juice of 2 limes
- 2 cloves garlic, minced
- 2 teaspoons honey
- 1 teaspoon smoked paprika
- Salt and black pepper, to taste
- Fresh parsley, chopped, for garnish
- Lemon wedges for serving

INSTRUCTIONS:

1. Ensure the shrimp are peeled and deveined. Pat them dry with paper towels.
2. Combine the olive oil, lemon zest, lemon juice, minced garlic, honey, smoked paprika, salt, and black pepper to make the marinade.
3. Put the shrimp in a shallow dish or resealable plastic bag. Pour the citrus marinade over the shrimp, ensuring they are well-coated. Let them marinate in the refrigerator for at least 15-30 minutes.
4. On medium-high heat, preheat a grill or grill pan.
5. Thread the marinated shrimp onto skewers, leaving space between each shrimp.
6. Shrimp skewers should be cooked on each side for two to three minutes or until they are opaque and have grill marks.
7. The shrimp are done when they turn pink and opaque. Be cautious not to overcook them to maintain their tenderness.

Nutritional Information (per serving):

Calories: 2256 | Fat: 112.5g | Saturated Fat: 18.1g | Cholesterol: 1264mg | Sodium: 1552mg | Carbohydrate: 188g | Fiber: 35.9g | Protein: 157.7g

NOTES:

- Adjust the honey and citrus levels based on your desired sweetness and tanginess.
- Serve over a bed of quinoa or a salad for a light and refreshing meal.

_____
_____
_____
_____

4.6 Mediterranean Chicken Skewers with Tzatziki

Preparation time	Cooking time	Servings
20 minutes	15 minutes	2

INGREDIENTS:

For Chicken Skewers:

- 2 boneless, skinless chicken breasts (about 12 oz or 340g total), cut into bite-sized cubes
- 2 tablespoons (30ml) olive oil
- 2 teaspoons dried oregano
- 2 teaspoons dried thyme
- 2 teaspoons smoked paprika
- 2 cloves garlic, minced
- Salt and black pepper, to taste
- Cherry tomatoes, for skewering
- Red onion, for skewering

For Tzatziki:

- 1/2 cup (120g) Greek yogurt
- 1/2 cucumber, finely diced
- 2 cloves garlic, minced
- 2 teaspoons fresh dill, chopped
- 2 teaspoons lemon juice
- Salt and black pepper, to taste

INSTRUCTIONS:

1. Mix olive oil, dried oregano, dried thyme, smoked paprika, minced garlic, salt, and black pepper in a bowl to create the marinade.
2. When adding the chicken cubes to the marinade, coat them thoroughly. Let them marinate for at least 15-30 minutes.
3. To make the tzatziki sauce, take another dish and mix Greek yogurt, finely sliced cucumber, minced garlic, chopped fresh dill, lemon juice, salt, and black pepper. Once fully combined, chill until ready to serve.
4. On medium-high heat, preheat a grill or grill pan.
5. Thread the marinated chicken cubes, cherry tomatoes, and red onion onto skewers, alternating the ingredients.
6. Grill the chicken skewers for about 3-4 minutes per side or until the chicken is cooked and has grill marks.
7. Ensure the chicken is no longer pink in the center and the juices run clear.

Nutritional Information (per serving):

Calories: 3582 | Fat: 176.8g | Saturated Fat: 35.1g | Cholesterol: 535mg | Sodium: 913mg | Carbohydrate: 352.4g | Fiber: 153.3g | Protein: 253.1g

NOTES:

- Customize the skewers with additional vegetables like bell peppers or zucchini.
- Drizzle extra tzatziki over the skewers for added flavor.

_____
_____
_____
_____

4.7 Blackened Tilapia with Mango Salsa

Preparation time	Cooking time	Servings
15 minutes	10 minutes	2

INGREDIENTS:

For Blackened Tilapia:
- 2 tilapia fillets (about 12 oz or 340g total)
- 2 teaspoons smoked paprika
- 1 teaspoon dried thyme
- 1 teaspoon onion powder
- 1 teaspoon garlic powder
- 1/2 tsp cayenne (adjust according to taste)
- To taste, add salt and black pepper.
- 2 tablespoons (30ml) olive oil

For Mango Salsa:
- 1 ripe mango, diced
- 1/2 red onion, finely chopped
- 1 red bell pepper, diced
- 2 tablespoons (30ml) fresh lime juice
- 2 tablespoons (30ml) fresh cilantro, chopped
- Salt and black pepper, to taste

INSTRUCTIONS:

1. Mix smoked paprika, dried thyme, onion powder, garlic powder, cayenne pepper, salt, and black pepper in a small bowl to create the blackening seasoning.
2. Pat the tilapia fillet dry with paper towels. Rub the blackening seasoning over both sides of the tilapia fillet, ensuring it's well-coated.
3. Olive oil should shimmer when heated in a skillet over medium-high heat.
4. Carefully place the seasoned tilapia fillet in the hot skillet. Cook for 3-4 minutes per side or until the tilapia is cooked through and has a blackened crust.
5. Prepare Mango Salsa:
6. Combine diced mango, finely chopped red onion, diced red bell pepper, fresh lime juice, chopped cilantro, salt, and black pepper in a bowl. Mix well to create the mango salsa.
7. Place the blackened tilapia on a plate and top it with a generous scoop of mango salsa.

Nutritional Information (per serving):

Calories: 2247 | Fat: 121.6g | Saturated Fat: 20.3g | Cholesterol: 292mg | Sodium: 19752mg | Carbohydrate: 205g | Fiber: 75.9g | Protein: 151.2g

NOTES:
- Adjust the cayenne pepper in the blackening seasoning based on your spice preference.
- Serve the blackened tilapia with rice or quinoa for a complete meal.

_____
_____
_____
_____

4.8 Balsamic Glazed Chicken Thighs

Preparation time	Cooking time	Servings
15 minutes	25 minutes	2

INGREDIENTS:

- 4 bone-in, skin-on chicken thighs
- Salt and black pepper, to taste
- 2 tablespoons (30ml) olive oil
- 4 cloves garlic, minced
- 1/2 cup (120ml) balsamic vinegar
- 2 tablespoons (30ml) honey
- 2 teaspoons Dijon mustard
- Fresh parsley, chopped, for garnish

INSTRUCTIONS:

1. Using paper towels, pat dry the chicken thighs. Add a sufficient amount of salt and black pepper to them.
2. Preheat the oven to 375°F (190°C).
3. Heat the olive oil in an oven-safe skillet to a medium-high temperature. Sear the chicken thighs, skin-side down, until golden brown (about 3-4 minutes).
4. Mix minced garlic, balsamic vinegar, honey, and Dijon mustard in a small bowl to create the glaze.
5. Pour the balsamic glaze over the seared chicken thighs, ensuring they are coated evenly.
6. When the chicken's skin is crispy and its internal temperature reaches 165°F (74°C), remove the pan from the oven and bake it for 25 to 30 minutes.
7. When you pierce the chicken with a fork, it should be cooked through because the juices should run clear.

Nutritional Information (per serving):

Calories: 1982 | Fat: 117.6g | Saturated Fat: 20.5g | Cholesterol: 145mg | Sodium: 1347mg | Carbohydrate: 189.7g | Fiber: 22.6g | Protein: 72.7g

NOTES:

- For extra flavor, marinate the chicken thighs in the balsamic glaze for 15-30 minutes before cooking.
- Serve with a side salad or your favorite roasted vegetables.

_____
_____
_____
_____

4.9 Spicy Chickpea and Turkey Lettuce Wraps

Preparation time	Cooking time	Servings
20 minutes	15 minutes	2

INGREDIENTS:

- 1 cup (240g) ground turkey
- 1 cup (240g) canned chickpeas, drained and rinsed
- 2 tablespoons (30ml) olive oil
- 1/2 cup (120ml) tomato sauce
- 2 teaspoons chili powder
- 1 teaspoon cumin
- 1/2 teaspoon smoked paprika
- Salt and black pepper, to taste
- Iceberg or butter lettuce leaves for wrapping
- Toppings: diced tomatoes, avocado, cilantro, lime wedges

INSTRUCTIONS:

1. The ground turkey should be browned and thoroughly cooked in a skillet over medium heat.
2. Add the canned chickpeas to the skillet with the cooked turkey and stir to combine.
3. Sprinkle chili powder, cumin, smoked paprika, salt, and black pepper over the turkey and chickpea mixture. Stir well to coat the ingredients with the spices evenly.
4. Mix tomato sauce into the skillet with the turkey and chickpeas. Allow it to simmer for 5-7 minutes until the flavors meld.
5. Wash and separate lettuce leaves, creating cups for the filling.
6. Spoon the spicy chickpea and turkey mixture into the lettuce cups.
7. Top the wraps with diced tomatoes, avocado slices, cilantro, and a squeeze of lime juice.

Nutritional Information (per serving):

Calories: 1668 | Fat: 133.1g | Saturated Fat: 18.8g | Cholesterol: 51mg | Sodium: 20680mg | Carbohydrate: 124.4g | Fiber: 58.5g | Protein: 49g

NOTES:

- Customize the spice level by adjusting the amount of chili powder.
- You can eat these wraps cold or warm.

CHAPTER 5: NUTRIENT-PACKED SIDES

These nutrient-packed side dishes are designed to complement your main courses while providing a wealth of vitamins, minerals, and antioxidants. Enjoy the vibrant and wholesome flavors!

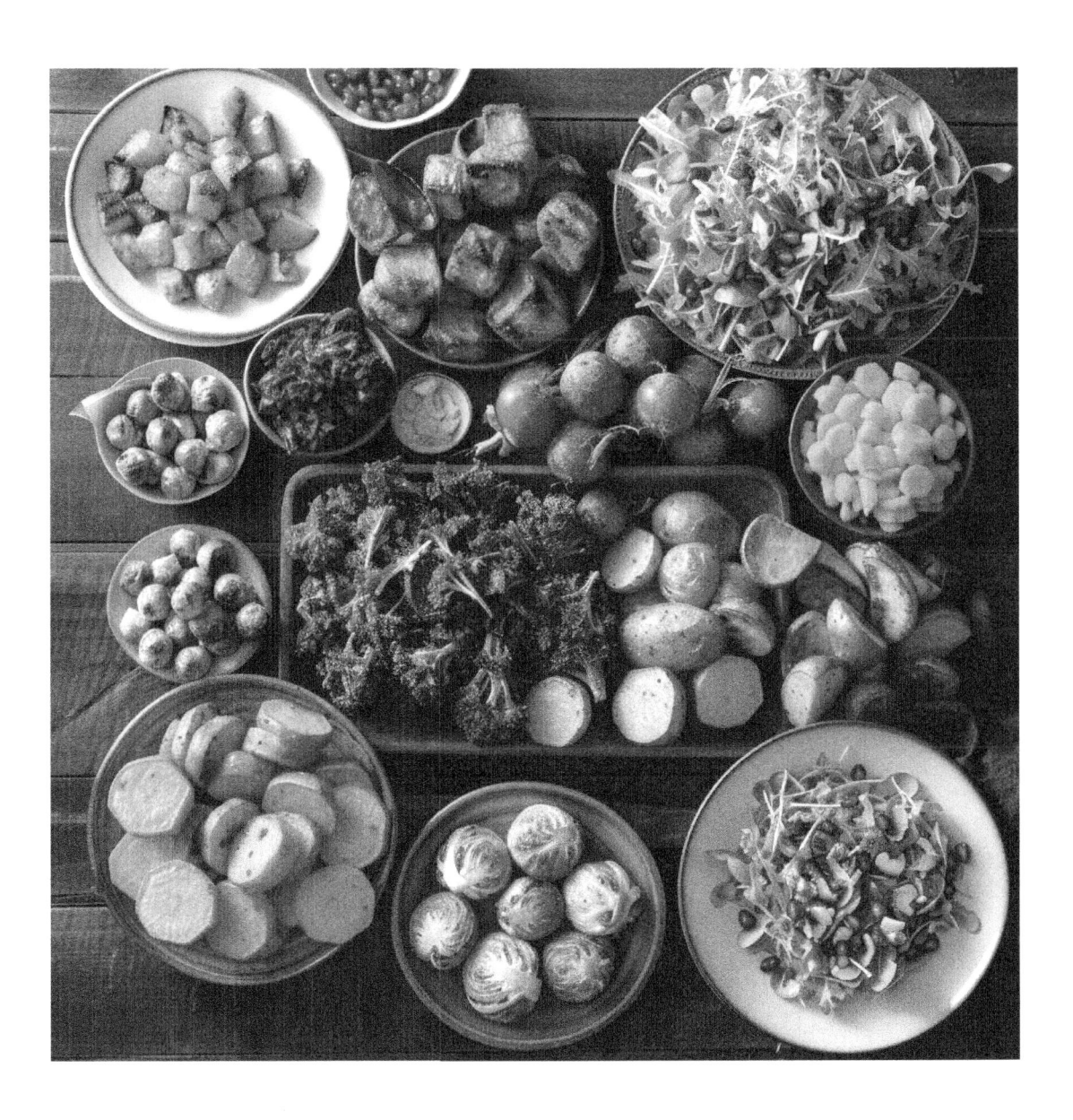

5.1 Garlic Lemon Roasted Brussels Sprouts

Preparation time	Cooking time	Servings
15 minutes	25 minutes	2

INGREDIENTS:

- 2 cups (300g) Brussels sprouts, trimmed and halved
- 4 tablespoons (60ml) olive oil
- 4 cloves garlic, minced
- Zest of 2 lemons
- 2 tablespoons (30ml) fresh lemon juice
- Salt and black pepper, to taste
- Optional: Grated Parmesan cheese for garnish
- Fresh parsley, chopped, for garnish

INSTRUCTIONS:

1. Preheat the oven to 400°F (200°C).
2. Trim the ends of the Brussels sprouts, cut them in half, and place them in a bowl.
3. Olive oil, minced garlic, lemon zest, and lemon juice should all be combined in a small basin. Mix well.
4. Drizzle the garlic lemon mixture over the Brussels sprouts, tossing them to ensure an even coating.
5. Season the Brussels sprouts with salt and black pepper, adjusting to taste.
6. On a baking sheet, arrange the Brussels sprouts in a single layer. Roast in a preheated oven for 20 to 25 minutes or until the edges are crispy and golden brown.
7. In the final five minutes of roasting, sprinkle grated Parmesan cheese over the Brussels sprouts if preferred.

Nutritional Information (per serving):

Calories: 2113 | Fat: 189.2g | Saturated Fat: 27.8g | Cholesterol: 0mg | Sodium: 19486mg | Carbohydrate: 112.5g | Fiber: 10g | Protein: 18.4g

NOTES:

- For the best tenderness, adjust the roasting time according to the size of the Brussels sprouts.
- Customize with your favorite herbs or additional seasonings.

_____
_____
_____
_____

5.2 Quinoa and Kale Stuffed Bell Peppers

Preparation time	Cooking time	Servings
20 minutes	30 minutes	2

INGREDIENTS:

- 4 bell peppers, halved and seeds removed
- 1 cup (180g) quinoa, cooked
- 2 cups (100g) kale, finely chopped
- 1/2 cup (50g) red onion, finely chopped
- 2 cloves garlic, minced
- 1/2 cup (60g) cherry tomatoes, diced
- 4 tablespoons (60ml) olive oil
- 2 teaspoons ground cumin
- 1 teaspoon smoked paprika
- Salt and black pepper, to taste
- 1/2 cup (60g) feta cheese, crumbled (optional)
- Fresh parsley, chopped, for garnish

INSTRUCTIONS:

1. Preheat the oven to 375°F (190°C).
2. After removing the seeds and cutting the bell peppers in half lengthwise, put them in a baking dish.
3. Cook quinoa according to package instructions if not already cooked.
4. In a skillet over medium heat, heat olive oil. Add chopped red onion and minced garlic, sautéing until softened.
5. Stir in chopped kale and diced cherry tomatoes, cooking until the kale wilts.
6. Add ground cumin, smoked paprika, salt, and black pepper to the skillet. Mix well.
7. Combine the sautéed vegetable mixture with cooked quinoa, ensuring it's well-mixed.
8. Press the quinoa and kale mixture into each half of the bell pepper.
9. Bake the bell peppers in a preheated oven for 25 to 30 minutes or until they are soft.
10. If using feta cheese, sprinkle it over the stuffed bell peppers during the last 5 minutes of baking.
11. Garnish with chopped fresh parsley before serving.

Nutritional Information (per serving):

Calories: 2804 | Fat: 227g | Saturated Fat: 34g | Cholesterol: 22mg | Sodium: 585mg | Carbohydrate: 205.6g | Fiber: 55.2g | Protein: 55g

NOTES:

- Feel free to customize the filling with your favorite vegetables or herbs.
- For added taste, add a dollop of Greek yogurt or a drizzle of balsamic glaze.

_____
_____
_____
_____

5.3 Sweet Potato and Black Bean Skillet

Preparation time	Cooking time	Servings
15 minutes	20 minutes	2

INGREDIENTS:

- 2 small sweet potatoes (about 400g total), peeled and diced
- 1 cup (180g) black beans, cooked and drained
- 1/2 cup (60g) red bell pepper, diced
- 1/2 cup (60g) red onion, finely chopped
- 2 cloves garlic, minced
- 2 tablespoons (30ml) olive oil
- 1 teaspoon ground cumin
- 1 teaspoon smoked paprika
- Salt and black pepper, to taste
- Fresh cilantro, chopped, for garnish
- Optional toppings: avocado slices, Greek yogurt

INSTRUCTIONS:

1. In a skillet over medium heat, add olive oil. Add diced sweet potatoes and sauté until slightly tender, about 5-7 minutes.
2. Add minced garlic, red onion, and diced bell pepper to the skillet. Continue cooking until the vegetables are softened.
3. Sprinkle ground cumin, smoked paprika, salt, and black pepper over the sweet potato and vegetable mixture. Mix well.
4. Stir in the cooked and drained black beans, ensuring even distribution.
5. To properly cook the sweet potatoes and enable the flavors to mingle, give the skillet another 5 to 7 minutes of cooking.
6. Taste and adjust the seasoning if needed.
7. Garnish the skillet with fresh cilantro. Optionally, serve with avocado slices and a dollop of Greek yogurt.

Nutritional Information (per serving):

Calories: 1621 | Fat: 112.7g | Saturated Fat: 15.5g | Cholesterol: 0mg | Sodium: 19536mg | Carbohydrate: 152.1g | Fiber: 40.8g | Protein: 38.5g

NOTES:

- Customize with your favorite toppings or additional spices.
- Serve over rice or quinoa, or enjoy it on its own.

5.4 Broccoli Almond Crunch Salad

Preparation time	Cooking time	Servings
15 minutes	-	2

INGREDIENTS:

- 2 cups (300g) broccoli florets, blanched and chopped
- 4 tablespoons (40g) almonds, sliced
- 4 tablespoons (60g) dried cranberries
- 1/2 cup (60g) red onion, finely chopped
- 4 tablespoons (60ml) Greek yogurt
- 2 tablespoons (30ml) apple cider vinegar
- 2 teaspoons honey
- Salt and black pepper, to taste
- Optional: Crumbled feta cheese for garnish

INSTRUCTIONS:

1. Broccoli florets should be blanched in boiling water for two to three minutes or until tender. Spoon over into ice water to halt cooking immediately. Dice into little pieces.
2. Toast the nut slices in a dry pan over medium heat until aromatic and golden brown. Keep a close eye to prevent burning.
3. Combine chopped broccoli, toasted almonds, dried cranberries, and finely chopped red onion in a bowl.
4. To create the dressing, combine Greek yogurt, honey, apple cider vinegar, salt, and black pepper in a small bowl.
5. After you've poured the dressing over the broccoli mixture, toss to coat every piece of broccoli.
6. After tasting the salad, taste and adjust the salt and pepper.
7. Feel free to top the salad with crumbled feta cheese for an added taste boost.

Nutritional Information (per serving):

Calories: 1786 | Fat: 104.4g | Saturated Fat: 10.6g | Cholesterol: 10mg | Sodium: 19490mg | Carbohydrate: 161.4g | Fiber: 35.6g | Protein: 65.8g

NOTES:

- Add tofu or grilled chicken to increase the protein content.
- Customize with your favorite nuts or seeds.

_____
_____
_____
_____

5.5 Spinach and Mushroom Quiche with Whole Wheat Crust

Preparation time	Cooking time	Servings
20 minutes	40 minutes	2

INGREDIENTS:

For Whole Wheat Crust:

- 1 cup (120g) whole wheat flour
- 4 tablespoons (60g) unsalted butter, cold and diced
- 4 tablespoons (60ml) ice-cold water
- A pinch of salt

For Quiche Filling:

- 1 cup (100g) spinach, chopped
- 1/2 cup (60g) mushrooms, sliced
- 1/2 cup (60g) red onion, finely chopped
- 2 cloves garlic, minced
- 2 teaspoons olive oil
- 4 eggs
- 1/2 cup (120ml) milk (any type)
- Salt and black pepper, to taste
- 4 tablespoons (60g) feta cheese, crumbled

INSTRUCTIONS:

For Whole Wheat Crust:

1. In a bowl, combine whole wheat flour and a pinch of salt. Toss in the chilled, chopped butter and massage it with your fingertips until the mixture looks like coarse crumbs.
2. Add ice-cold water, one tablespoon, and mix until the dough comes together. Form it into a disc, wrap it in plastic wrap, and refrigerate for 30 minutes.
3. Turn the oven on to 375°F, or 190°C. Roll out the chilled dough on a surface dusted with flour and transfer it to a small tart or quiche pan. Press it into the pan and trim the excess dough.
4. The crust lined with parchment paper can be filled with dried beans or pie weights. After 15 minutes of blind baking and removing the weights, bake the crust for a further 5 minutes or until it turns golden brown.

For Quiche Filling:

1. Warm up the olive oil in a pan over medium heat. Sauté chopped spinach, sliced mushrooms, red onion, and minced garlic until vegetables are softened. Set aside.
2. Whisk together eggs, milk, black pepper, and salt in a bowl.
3. Spread the sautéed vegetable mixture over the pre-baked crust. Cover the veggies with the egg and milk mixture. Sprinkle crumbled feta cheese on top.
4. Bake in the oven for 20-25 minutes or until the quiche is set and the top is golden brown.

Nutritional Information (per serving):

Calories: 3418 | Fat: 319.8g | Saturated Fat: 152.7g | Cholesterol: 1354mg | Sodium: 23115mg | Carbohydrate: 87.3g | Fiber: 5.3g | Protein: 70.1g

NOTES:
- Add your preferred cheese and vegetables to the filling.
- Enjoy this quiche for breakfast, brunch, or a light dinner.

_____
_____
_____
_____

5.6 Avocado Cilantro Lime Rice

Preparation time	Cooking time	Servings
10 minutes	15 minutes	2

INGREDIENTS:
- 1 cup (180g) cooked brown rice
- 1 ripe avocado, diced
- 4 tablespoons (60g) fresh cilantro, chopped
- 2 tablespoons (30ml) lime juice
- 2 teaspoons lime zest
- 2 tablespoons (30ml) extra-virgin olive oil
- Salt and black pepper, to taste
- Red pepper flakes, for an optional spicy kick

INSTRUCTIONS:
1. Ensure that the brown rice is cooked and ready for use.
2. Dice half a ripe avocado.
3. Cooked brown rice, diced avocado, chopped fresh cilantro, lime zest, and lime juice should all be combined in a bowl.
4. Drizzle extra-virgin olive oil over the mixture.
5. Season with salt and black pepper to taste. Add red pepper flakes if you desire a bit of heat.
6. Gently toss the ingredients until well combined, ensuring the avocado is evenly distributed.
7. Serve the Avocado Cilantro Lime Rice as a side dish or a light, refreshing main.

Nutritional Information (per serving):

Calories: 1201 | Fat: 105.8g | Saturated Fat: 15.7g | Cholesterol: 0mg | Sodium: 19484mg | Carbohydrate: 74.1g | Fiber: 21.7g | Protein: 10.9g

NOTES:
- Customize with additional herbs or vegetables such as diced tomatoes or red onion.
- Squeeze additional lime juice if you prefer a more citrusy flavor.

_____
_____
_____

5.7 Roasted Asparagus with Parmesan and Lemon

Preparation time	Cooking time	Servings
10 minutes	15 minutes	2

INGREDIENTS:

- 2 bunches (about 300g) fresh asparagus, tough ends trimmed
- 2 tablespoons (30ml) olive oil
- Zest of 2 lemons
- 2 tablespoons (30ml) fresh lemon juice
- 4 tablespoons (40g) Parmesan cheese, grated
- Salt and black pepper, to taste
- Red pepper flakes, for an optional spicy kick

INSTRUCTIONS:

1. Preheat the oven to 400°F (200°C).
2. Snip off the asparagus spears' rough ends.
3. Place the asparagus on a baking sheet. Make sure the asparagus is evenly covered, and drizzle some olive oil over them.
4. Sprinkle lemon zest over the asparagus, and squeeze fresh lemon juice.
5. Season with salt and black pepper to taste. Add red pepper flakes if you desire a bit of spice.
6. Toss the asparagus on the baking sheet to evenly coat it with the olive oil, lemon, and seasonings.
7. Roast the asparagus for 12 to 15 minutes in a preheated oven or until it is crisp but still soft.
8. While the asparagus is still warm, sprinkle grated Parmesan cheese over the top.

Nutritional Information (per serving):

Calories: 1656 | Fat: 145.8g | Saturated Fat: 44.4g | Cholesterol: 143mg | Sodium: 21274mg | Carbohydrate: 43.4g | Fiber: 17.2g | Protein: 74.4g

NOTES:

- Adjust roasting time based on the thickness of asparagus spears.
- Customize with your favorite herbs or additional seasonings.

5.8 Cauliflower and Chickpea Curry

Preparation time	Cooking time	Servings
20 minutes	25 minutes	2

INGREDIENTS:

- 2 cups (300g) cauliflower florets
- 1 cup (170g) cooked chickpeas
- 1 cup (240ml) coconut milk
- 1/2 cup (120ml) vegetable broth
- 2 tablespoons (30ml) olive oil
- 1 onion, finely chopped
- 2 cloves garlic, minced
- 2 teaspoons ginger, grated
- 2 tablespoons (24g) curry powder
- 1 teaspoon ground cumin
- 1 teaspoon ground coriander
- 1/2 teaspoon turmeric powder
- 1/2 teaspoon cayenne pepper (adjust according to taste)
- Salt and black pepper, to taste
- Fresh cilantro leaves for garnish
- Cooked brown rice or quinoa for serving

INSTRUCTIONS:

1. Warm up the olive oil in a big skillet over medium heat. Add finely chopped onion, minced garlic, and grated ginger. Sauté until the onions are translucent.
2. Add curry powder, cumin, coriander, turmeric powder, and cayenne pepper to the skillet. Stir well to coat the aromatics with the spices.
3. Add cauliflower florets and cooked chickpeas to the skillet. Stir to combine with the spice mixture.
4. Add the veggie broth and coconut milk to the skillet. Stir to combine, ensuring the cauliflower and chickpeas are coated in the flavorful sauce.
5. Once the cauliflower is soft and the flavors have combined, reduce the heat and simmer the curry for 15 to 20 minutes.
6. Season with salt and black pepper to taste. Adjust the spice level if needed.

Nutritional Information (per serving):

Calories: 2515 | Fat: 148.4g | Saturated Fat: 31.2g | Cholesterol: 0mg | Sodium: 19737mg | Carbohydrate: 297.6g | Fiber: 81.6g | Protein: 60.7g

NOTES:

- Customize with additional vegetables such as spinach or bell peppers.
- For brightness, squeeze in some fresh lemon juice.

_____
_____
_____
_____

5.9 Mediterranean Couscous Salad

Preparation time	Cooking time	Servings
15 minutes	10 minutes	2

INGREDIENTS:

- 1 cup (180g) couscous
- 1 cup (240ml) vegetable broth or water
- 1/2 cup (80g) cherry tomatoes, halved
- 1/2 cup (80g) cucumber, diced
- 1/2 cup (80g) red bell pepper, diced
- 4 tablespoons (60g) red onion, finely chopped
- 4 tablespoons (60g) Kalamata olives, pitted and sliced
- 2 tablespoons (30ml) extra-virgin olive oil
- 2 tablespoons (30ml) balsamic vinegar
- 1 teaspoon dried oregano
- Salt and black pepper, to taste
- Feta cheese crumbles for garnish (optional)
- Fresh parsley, chopped, for garnish

INSTRUCTIONS:

1. In a small saucepan, bring vegetable broth or water to a boil. Add couscous, cover, and remove from heat. After five minutes, use a fork to fluff it up.
2. Let the couscous cool until it reaches room temperature.
3. Cool couscous, cherry tomatoes, cucumber, red bell pepper, red onion, and Kalamata olives should all be combined in a big bowl.
4. Mix the dried oregano, balsamic vinegar, extra virgin olive oil, salt, and black pepper in a small bowl.
5. Drizzle the dressing over the couscous and vegetables. Toss until everything is well coated.
6. Garnish with feta cheese crumbles (if using) and fresh parsley.

Nutritional Information (per serving):

Calories: 1498 | Fat: 120.8g | Saturated Fat: 17.7g | Cholesterol: 0mg | Sodium: 21310mg | Carbohydrate: 107.4g | Fiber: 35.4g | Protein: 17.5g

NOTES:

- Customize with your favorite Mediterranean ingredients like artichoke hearts or roasted red peppers.
- Add grilled chicken or chickpeas for added protein.

CHAPTER 6: WHOLE-GRAIN WONDERS

These whole-grain marvels are high in fiber, vitamins, minerals, and deliciousness. Enjoy the diverse and wholesome goodness of whole grains!

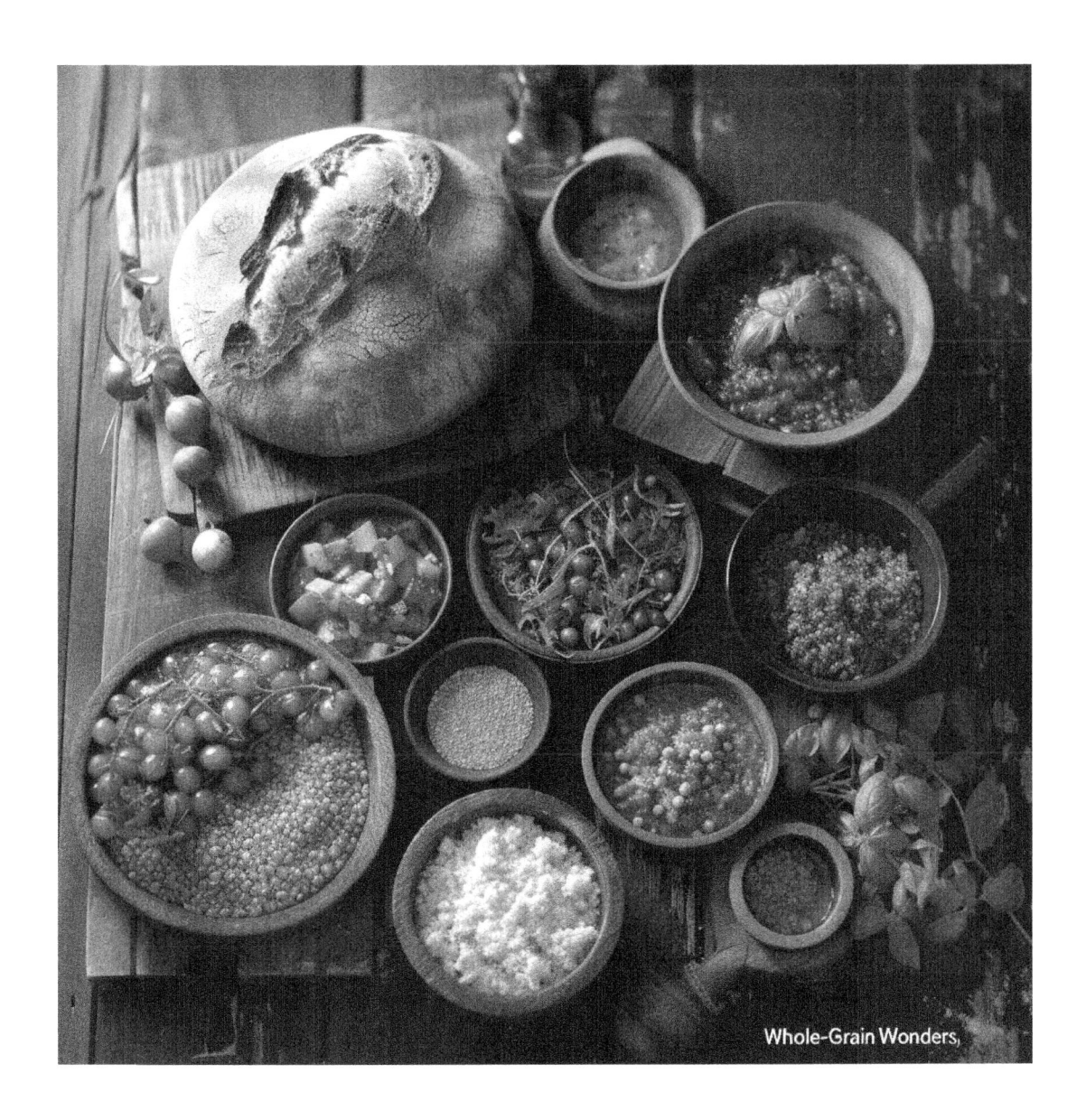

6.1 Farro Salad with Roasted Vegetables and Feta

Preparation time	Cooking time	Servings
20 minutes	25 minutes	2

INGREDIENTS:

- 1 cup (180g) farro, cooked
- 1 cup (150g) cherry tomatoes, halved
- 1/2 cup (80g) red bell pepper, diced
- 1/2 cup (80g) zucchini, diced
- 1/2 cup (80g) red onion, thinly sliced
- 4 tablespoons (60g) feta cheese, crumbled
- 2 tablespoons (30ml) extra-virgin olive oil
- 2 tablespoons (30ml) balsamic vinegar
- 2 teaspoons dried oregano
- Salt and black pepper, to taste
- Fresh basil, chopped, for garnish

INSTRUCTIONS:

1. Cook Farro: Ensure that the farro is cooked and ready for use.
2. Preheat the oven to 400°F (200°C). Toss cherry tomatoes, red bell pepper, zucchini, and thinly sliced red onion with olive oil, balsamic vinegar, dried oregano, salt, and black pepper. The veggies should be roasted for 15 to 20 minutes or until they are soft and have a hint of caramel.
3. Combine the cooked farro, roasted vegetables, and crumbled feta cheese in a bowl. Mix well.
4. Taste and adjust the seasoning if needed. Drizzle with additional olive oil or balsamic vinegar if desired.
5. Garnish the Farro Salad with Roasted Vegetables and Feta with fresh chopped basil.

Nutritional Information (per serving):

Calories: 1828 | Fat: 146.4g | Saturated Fat: 45.9g | Cholesterol: 178mg | Sodium: 21664mg | Carbohydrate: 110g | Fiber: 47.3g | Protein: 46.9g

NOTES:

- For added freshness, toss in a handful of baby spinach or arugula.
- Customize with your favorite roasted vegetables like eggplant or bell peppers.

6.2 Quinoa and Black Bean Stuffed Peppers

Preparation time	Cooking time	Servings
20 minutes	40 minutes	2

INGREDIENTS:

- 4 large bell peppers, halved and seeds removed
- 1 cup (180g) cooked quinoa
- 1 cup (200g) black beans, cooked or canned (rinsed and drained)
- 1/2 cup (120g) corn kernels (fresh, frozen, or canned)
- 1/2 cup (80g) red onion, finely chopped
- 1 cup (230g) tomato sauce
- 2 teaspoons ground cumin
- 1 teaspoon chili powder
- 1 teaspoon paprika
- Salt and black pepper, to taste
- 1/2 cup (60g) shredded cheddar cheese (optional)
- Fresh cilantro, chopped, for garnish
- Lime wedges for serving

INSTRUCTIONS:

1. Preheat your oven to 375°F (190°C).
2. Trim the bell peppers of their seeds and membranes by cutting them in half lengthwise.
3. Ensure that the quinoa is cooked and ready for use.
4. Combine cooked quinoa, black beans, corn, red onion, tomato sauce, ground cumin, chili powder, paprika, salt, and black pepper in a bowl. Mix well to incorporate all ingredients.
5. Fill each half of a bell pepper with a spoonful of the quinoa and black bean mixture, gently pressing down to compact the filling.
6. The filled peppers should be put in a roasting tray. Garnish with shredded cheddar cheese if you'd like. Once the peppers are soft, bake the dish covered with foil for 25 to 30 minutes.
7. Take it out of the oven and top it with chopped fresh cilantro.

Nutritional Information (per serving):

Calories: 1263 | Fat: 50.3g | Saturated Fat: 10g | Cholesterol: 26mg | Sodium: 20504mg | Carbohydrate: 193.3g | Fiber: 62.9g | Protein: 60g

NOTES:

- Make the stuffing unique by adding your preferred spices or veggies.
- Drizzle with hot sauce, or add a dollop of Greek yogurt for extra flavor.

6.3 Brown Rice and Vegetable Stir-Fry

Preparation time	Cooking time	Servings
15 minutes	15 minutes	2

INGREDIENTS:

- 1 cup (180g) brown rice, cooked
- 1 cup (150g) broccoli florets
- 1 cup (120g) snap peas, trimmed
- 1 medium carrot, julienned
- 1/2 cup (80g) red bell pepper, thinly sliced
- 4 tablespoons (60g) corn kernels (fresh or frozen)
- 4 tablespoons (60ml) soy sauce
- 2 tablespoons (30ml) sesame oil
- 2 tablespoons (30ml) rice vinegar
- 2 teaspoons fresh ginger, grated
- 2 cloves garlic, minced
- 2 green onions, chopped
- Sesame seeds, for garnish (optional)

INSTRUCTIONS:

1. Cook Brown Rice: Ensure the brown rice is cooked and ready for use.
2. Heat some sesame oil over medium-high heat in a work or large skillet. Add broccoli, snap peas, julienned carrot, sliced red bell pepper, and corn. Stir-fry for 3-5 minutes until vegetables are slightly tender but crisp.
3. Grated ginger, minced garlic, rice vinegar, sesame oil, and soy sauce should all be combined in a small bowl.
4. Add the cooked brown rice to the stir-fried vegetables.
5. Over the rice and veggies, drizzle the prepared sauce. Stir to coat evenly.
6. Let the rice absorb the sauce and the flavors to mingle by cooking for two to three minutes.
7. Garnish the stir-fry with chopped green onions and sesame seeds (if using).

Nutritional Information (per serving):

Calories: 2408 | Fat: 137g | Saturated Fat: 20.7g | Cholesterol: 0mg | Sodium: 11447mg | Carbohydrate: 252g | Fiber: 40.3g | Protein: 57.3g

NOTES:

- Customize with your favorite vegetables, such as mushrooms, bell peppers, or baby corn.
- Add tofu, chicken, or shrimp for added protein.

6.4 Whole Wheat Mediterranean Pizza with Hummus Base

Preparation time	Cooking time	Servings
15 minutes	15 minutes	2

INGREDIENTS:

- 2 whole wheat pizza crusts (store-bought or homemade)
- 1/2 cup (120g) hummus (store-bought or homemade)
- 1 cup (150g) cherry tomatoes, halved
- 1/2 cup (80g) cucumber, thinly sliced
- 4 tablespoons (60g) Kalamata olives, pitted and sliced
- 4 tablespoons (60g) red onion, thinly sliced
- 1/2 cup (80g) feta cheese, crumbled
- 2 tablespoons (30ml) extra-virgin olive oil
- 2 teaspoons dried oregano
- Salt and black pepper, to taste
- Fresh parsley, chopped, for garnish

INSTRUCTIONS:

1. Preheat your oven as directed by the pizza crust's packaging or the recipe you produced at home.
2. Place the whole wheat pizza crust on a baking sheet or pizza stone.
3. Leave a thin border all the way around, and evenly cover the pizza crust with hummus.
4. Arrange cherry tomatoes, cucumber slices, Kalamata olives, and red onion on the hummus-covered crust.
5. Crumble feta cheese over the pizza.
6. Drizzle extra-virgin olive oil over the toppings.
7. Sprinkle dried oregano, salt, and black pepper to taste.
8. Bake your pizza crust according to the manufacturer's instructions or until the crust is brown and the toppings are well-cooked.

Nutritional Information (per serving):

Calories: 1782 | Fat: 136.1g | Saturated Fat: 23.7g | Cholesterol: 22mg | Sodium: 22246mg | Carbohydrate: 150.8g | Fiber: 57.3g | Protein: 28.7g

NOTES:

- Customize with additional Mediterranean toppings like artichoke hearts or roasted red peppers.
- Consider adding a handful of fresh arugula just before serving for extra freshness.

___
___
___
___

6.5 Spaghetti Squash Primavera

Preparation time	Cooking time	Servings
15 minutes	40 minutes	2

INGREDIENTS:

- 1 small spaghetti squash
- 1 cup (150g) cherry tomatoes, halved
- 1/2 cup (80g) yellow bell pepper, thinly sliced
- 1/2 cup (80g) zucchini, julienned
- 4 tablespoons (60g) red onion, finely chopped
- 2 cloves garlic, minced
- 4 tablespoons (60ml) olive oil
- 1/2 teaspoon dried thyme
- 1/2 teaspoon dried oregano
- Salt and black pepper, to taste
- 4 tablespoons (60g) Parmesan cheese, grated
- Fresh basil, chopped, for garnish

INSTRUCTIONS:

1. Preheat the oven to 400°F (200°C). Scoop out the seeds, cut the spaghetti squash in half lengthwise, and put the halves on a baking sheet. After adding a dab of olive oil, season with pepper and salt. Roast in the oven for about 40-45 minutes or until the flesh is fork-tender.
2. Allow the roasted spaghetti squash to cool slightly. Utilizing a fork, scrape the meat to form spaghetti-like strands. Transfer the strands to a bowl.
3. Add the olive oil to a pan and place over medium heat. Add minced garlic, cherry tomatoes, sliced yellow bell pepper, julienned zucchini, and chopped red onion. Vegetables should be sautéed for 5 to 7 minutes or until soft but bright.
4. Season the vegetables with dried thyme, oregano, salt, and black pepper. Toss to combine.
5. Add the roasted spaghetti squash strands to the skillet. Toss everything together until well combined.
6. Transfer the Spaghetti Squash Primavera to a serving plate. As a garnish, add some freshly chopped basil and top with grated Parmesan cheese.

Nutritional Information (per serving):

Calories: 2783 | Fat: 236.8g | Saturated Fat: 57.2g | Cholesterol: 143mg | Sodium: 1936mg | Carbohydrate: 131.9g | Fiber: 40.9g | Protein: 84.7g

NOTES:

- Customize with your favorite vegetables, like mushrooms or spinach.
- To serve, drizzle with a little olive oil or a squeeze of lemon.

6.6 Whole-grain Couscous with Lemon and Herbs

Preparation time	Cooking time	Servings
15 minutes	10 minutes	2

INGREDIENTS:

- 1 cup (180g) whole-grain couscous
- 2 cups (480ml) vegetable broth
- Zest of 1 lemon
- 2 tablespoons (30ml) fresh lemon juice
- 2 tablespoons (30ml) olive oil
- 2 cloves garlic, minced
- 2 tablespoons (30g) fresh parsley, chopped
- 2 tablespoons (30g) fresh mint, chopped
- Salt and black pepper, to taste

INSTRUCTIONS:

1. The vegetable broth should be brought to a boil in a saucepan. Stir in the whole-grain couscous, cover, and remove from heat. Let it sit for about 5 minutes or until the couscous absorbs the liquid.
2. To separate the grains, fluff the couscous using a fork.
3. Olive oil, fresh lemon juice, zest, minced garlic, chopped parsley, and chopped mint should all be combined in a small bowl.
4. Pour the lemon-herb dressing over the fluffed couscous. Gently toss to combine, ensuring the couscous is evenly coated.
5. Season the Whole-grain Couscous with Lemon and Herbs with salt and black pepper to taste. Adjust the seasoning as needed.
6. Garnish with additional chopped herbs and a lemon wedge if desired.

Nutritional Information (per serving):

Calories: 1209 | Fat: 102.2g | Saturated Fat: 15.2g | Cholesterol: 0mg | Sodium: 20080mg | Carbohydrate: 69.8g | Fiber: 16.6g | Protein: 19.4g

NOTES:

- Customize with your favorite herbs like cilantro or dill.
- Add in some toasted pine nuts or almonds for extra crunch.

6.7 Wild Rice Pilaf with Cranberries and Almonds

Preparation time	Cooking time	Servings
15 minutes	40 minutes	2

INGREDIENTS:

- 1 cup (180g) wild rice
- 2 cups (480ml) vegetable broth
- 1/2 cup (80g) dried cranberries
- 4 tablespoons (60g) almonds, sliced
- 2 tablespoons (30ml) olive oil
- 1/2 cup (80g) onion, finely chopped
- 2 cloves garlic, minced
- 1 teaspoon dried thyme
- Salt and black pepper, to taste
- Fresh parsley, chopped, for garnish

INSTRUCTIONS:

1. Rinse the wild rice under cold water. In a saucepan, combine the wild rice with vegetable broth. Once the wild rice is soft and has absorbed the liquid, lower the heat, cover it, and simmer it for 45 to 50 minutes.
2. Fluff the cooked wild rice using a fork and allow it to cool slightly.
3. In a dry skillet, toast the sliced almonds over medium heat until golden brown. Keep an eye on them to prevent burning.
4. Olive oil should be heated at a medium temperature in the same pan. Add finely chopped onion and minced garlic. Saute until the onion becomes translucent.
5. Combine the sautéed onion and garlic with the cooked wild rice in a skillet. Stir to combine.
6. Toss in the dried cranberries and toasted sliced almonds. Stir until evenly distributed.
7. Season the Wild Rice Pilaf with Cranberries and Almonds with dried thyme, salt, and black pepper. Adjust the seasoning to taste.
8. Garnish the pilaf with fresh chopped parsley.

Nutritional Information (per serving):

Calories: 2462 | Fat: 198.7g | Saturated Fat: 22.6g | Cholesterol: 0mg | Sodium: 19748mg | Carbohydrate: 150.3g | Fiber: 50.2g | Protein: 62.9g

NOTES:

- Customize with additional herbs or a squeeze of lemon juice for brightness.
- Add a handful of arugula or spinach for a fresh touch.

_____
_____
_____
_____

6.8 Bulgur and Chickpea Salad with Tahini Dressing

Preparation time	Cooking time	Servings
15 minutes	15 minutes	2

INGREDIENTS:

- 1 cup (180g) coarse bulgur
- 2 cups (480ml) boiling water
- 1 cup (170g) canned chickpeas, drained and rinsed
- 1/2 cup (80g) cucumber, diced
- 1/2 cup (80g) cherry tomatoes, halved
- 4 tablespoons (60g) red onion, finely chopped
- 2 tablespoons (30g) fresh parsley, chopped
- 2 tablespoons (30ml) olive oil
- 2 tablespoons (30ml) tahini
- 2 tablespoons (30ml) lemon juice
- 2 cloves garlic, minced
- Salt and black pepper, to taste

INSTRUCTIONS:

1. Place the coarse bulgur in a heatproof bowl. Pour boiling water over the bulgur, cover the bowl, and let it sit for about 15-20 minutes or until it absorbs the water and becomes tender.
2. Using a fork, fluff the cooked bulgur and let it cool.
3. To create the tahini dressing, combine the olive oil, tahini, lemon juice, minced garlic, salt, and black pepper in a small bowl.
4. The cooked bulgur, chickpeas, diced cucumber, cherry tomatoes, minced red onion, and fresh parsley should all be combined in a big bowl.
5. Pour the tahini dressing over the salad ingredients. Toss until everything is well coated.
6. If necessary, taste and add more salt and black pepper to the seasoning.

Nutritional Information (per serving):

Calories: 1916 | Fat: 152.6g | Saturated Fat: 22.2g | Cholesterol: 0mg | Sodium: 19614mg | Carbohydrate: 122.9g | Fiber: 30.8g | Protein: 40.9g

NOTES:

- Add your preferred vegetables, like olives or bell peppers, to personalize.
- Add a sprinkle of feta cheese for added richness.

_____
_____
_____
_____

6.9 Oat and Chia Seed Breakfast Bowl

Preparation time	Cooking time	Servings
10 minutes	Overnight or at least 4 hours for soaking.	2

INGREDIENTS:

- 1/2 cup (45g) rolled oats
- 2 tablespoons (20g) chia seeds
- 1/2 cup (120ml) almond milk (or any milk of your choice)
- 1/2 cup (120ml) Greek yogurt
- 1 tablespoon (15g) honey or maple syrup
- 1/2 teaspoon vanilla extract
- Fresh fruit for garnish, such as sliced mango, banana slices, or berries
- Nuts and seeds for garnishing, including almonds, chia seeds, or pumpkin seeds

INSTRUCTIONS:

1. Combine rolled oats, chia seeds, almond milk, Greek yogurt, honey or maple syrup, and vanilla extract in a bowl. For everything to be evenly blended, give it a good stir.
2. Place a lid on the bowl and place it in the refrigerator for at least 4 hours or overnight. This enables the liquids to seep into the oats and chia seeds, causing them to soften.
3. Before serving, stir the mixture to make it creamy and well combined.
4. Transfer the Oat and Chia Seed Breakfast Bowl to a serving dish. Top with your favorite fresh fruits and a sprinkle of nuts or seeds.
5. Optional: Drizzle with More Honey or Maple Syrup.

Nutritional Information (per serving):

Calories: 1764 | Fat: 77.7g | Saturated Fat: 18.5g | Cholesterol: 3mg | Sodium: 67mg | Carbohydrate: 211.6g | Fiber: 75.2g | Protein: 46.2g

NOTES:

- Experiment with different fruit combinations and nut toppings.
- Add a sprinkling of coconut flakes or a dash of cinnamon for added taste.

CHAPTER 7: SNACK ATTACK

These snack recipes are delicious and provide a good balance of nutrients to keep you energized between meals. Enjoy the satisfying and healthy snack options!

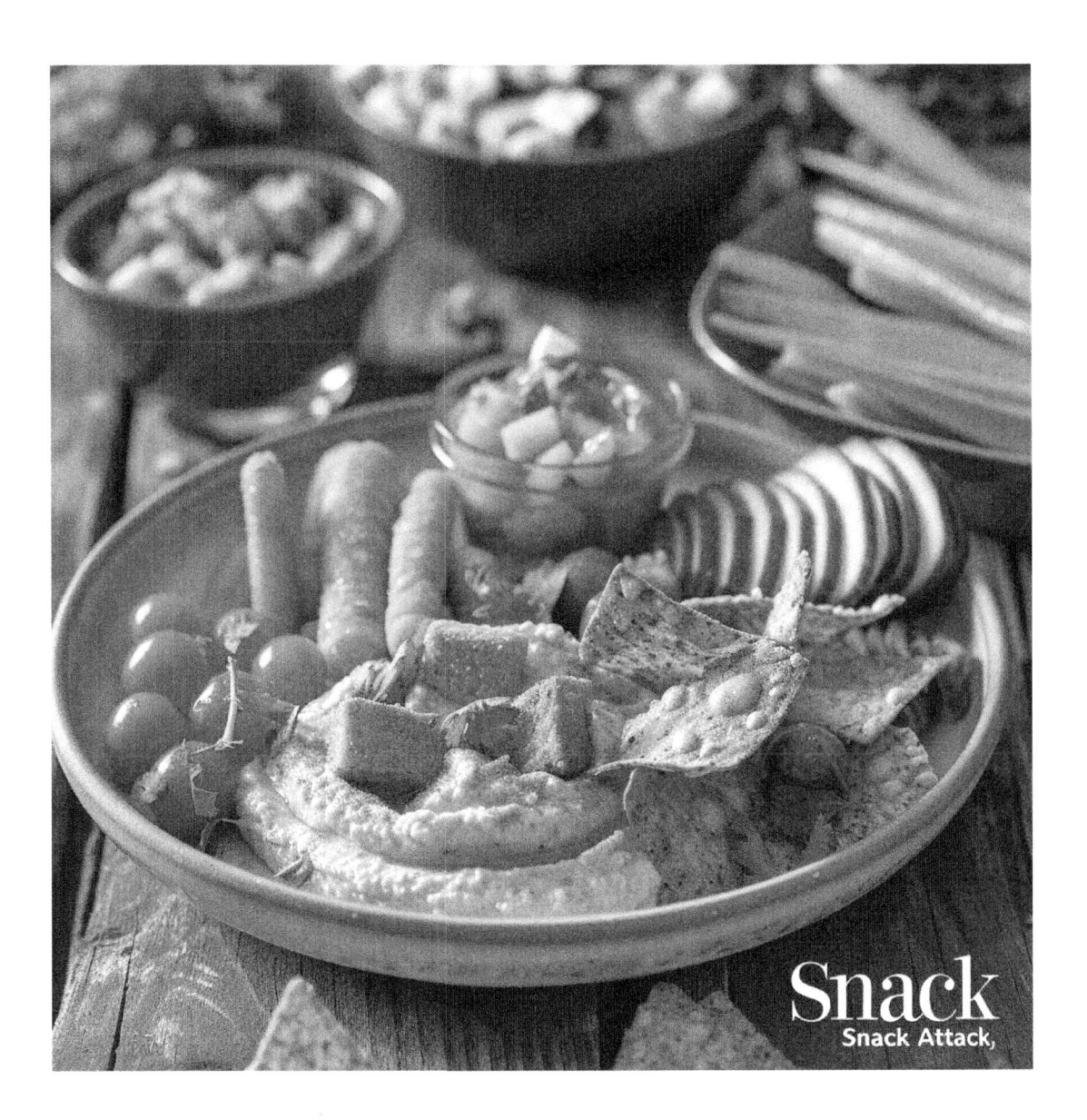

7.1 Trail Mix with Nuts and Dried Fruit

Preparation time	Cooking time	Servings
10 minutes	-	2

INGREDIENTS:

- 1/2 cup (60g) almonds
- 1/2 cup (60g) walnuts
- 1/2 cup (80g) dried cranberries
- 1/2 cup (80g) raisins
- 1/2 cup (60g) pumpkin seeds
- 1/2 cup (60g) dark chocolate chips (optional)
- 1/2 teaspoon ground cinnamon (optional)
- A pinch of salt (optional)

INSTRUCTIONS:

1. Mix almonds, walnuts, pumpkin seeds, and any other nuts or seeds of your choice in a bowl.
2. Add dried cranberries and raisins to the nut and seed mixture. Toss to combine.
3. If desired, include dark chocolate chips for a sweet touch. This is optional and can be adjusted based on your preference.
4. Sprinkle with Cinnamon and Salt (Optional): For added flavor, sprinkle ground cinnamon over the trail mix. Add a pinch of salt if you like a sweet-savory contrast.
5. Mix all the ingredients thoroughly, ensuring an even distribution of nuts, seeds, dried fruit, and any optional additions.

Nutritional Information (per serving):

Calories: 639 | Fat: 45.5g | Saturated Fat: 8.1g | Cholesterol: 0mg | Sodium: 19387mg | Carbohydrate: 51g | Fiber: 7.7g | Protein: 19.9g

NOTES:

- Customize the trail mix by adding your favorite nuts, seeds, or dried fruits.
- Adjust the quantity of chocolate chips or omit them based on your preference.

7.2 Guacamole with Baked Whole Wheat Tortilla Chips

Preparation time	Cooking time	Servings
15 minutes	10 minutes	2

Guacamole INGREDIENTS:

- 2 ripe avocados, peeled and pitted
- 1/2 cup (120g) red onion, finely diced
- 1 medium tomato, diced
- 1/2 cup (30g) fresh cilantro, chopped
- 1 lime, juiced
- 1 teaspoon garlic, minced
- Salt and pepper, to taste

Baked Whole Wheat Tortilla Chips INGREDIENTS:

- 2 whole wheat tortillas
- Olive oil spray
- Sea salt, to taste

INSTRUCTIONS:

For Guacamole:

1. In a bowl, mash the ripe avocado using a fork.
2. Add diced tomato, red onion, minced garlic, chopped cilantro, lime juice, and salt and pepper to the mashed avocado. Until the ingredients are uniformly blended, thoroughly mix everything.
3. Taste the guacamole and adjust the seasoning according to your preference. Add more lime juice, salt, or pepper if needed.
4. Cover the guacamole with plastic wrap and press it firmly onto the top to keep it from browning. Refrigerate until ready to serve.

For Baked Whole Wheat Tortilla Chips:

1. Preheat the oven to 350°F (180°C).
2. Cut the whole wheat tortilla into triangles or desired chip shapes.
3. Arrange the triangles of tortilla in a single layer on a baking sheet.
4. Lightly spray the tortilla triangles with olive oil. This aids in their oven-baking crispiness.
5. Sprinkle sea salt over the tortilla triangles for added flavor.
6. The chips should bake for 8 to 10 minutes in a preheated oven or until crispy and golden brown.
7. Allow the baked tortilla chips to cool before serving.

Nutritional Information (per serving):

Calories: 951 | Fat: 68.9g | Saturated Fat: 10.8g | Cholesterol: 0mg | Sodium: 39185mg | Carbohydrate: 82.2g | Fiber: 17.4g | Protein: 15.2g

NOTES:

- Feel free to add diced jalapeños for some heat.
- Customize the guacamole with additional ingredients like diced bell peppers or corn.

7.3 Greek Yogurt and Berry Parfait

Preparation time	Cooking time	Servings
10 minutes	-	2

INGREDIENTS:

- 1 cup (240g) Greek yogurt
- 1/2 cup (60g) granola
- 1 cup (140g) mixed berries (strawberries, blueberries, raspberries)
- 2 tablespoons (30g) honey or maple syrup (optional)
- Fresh mint leaves for garnish (optional)

INSTRUCTIONS:

1. Add half of the Greek yogurt to the bottom of a glass or serving dish.
2. Sprinkle a layer of granola over the Greek yogurt, creating a delicious and crunchy texture.
3. Place a layer of mixed berries over the granola, covering the surface evenly.
4. Repeat the layers by adding the remaining Greek yogurt, another layer of granola, and then the rest of the mixed berries.
5. If you desire added sweetness, drizzle honey or maple syrup over the top of the parfait. (Optional)
6. For a fresh touch, garnish the parfait with a few mint leaves. (Optional)
7. Serve the Greek Yogurt and Berry Parfait immediately to enjoy the contrast of creamy yogurt, crunchy granola, and the burst of flavors from the berries.

Nutritional Information (per serving):

Calories: 477 | Fat: 7.4g | Saturated Fat: 1.9g | Cholesterol: 3mg | Sodium: 42mg | Carbohydrate: 124.4g | Fiber: 7.4g | Protein: 11.2g

NOTES:

- Feel free to customize by adding nuts or seeds for extra crunch.
- Adjust the sweetness by varying the amount of honey or maple syrup.

_____
_____
_____
_____

7.4 Apple Slices with Almond Butter and Cinnamon

Preparation time	Cooking time	Servings
10 minutes	-	2

INGREDIENTS:

- 2 medium apples (e.g., Honeycrisp or Fuji), sliced
- 4 tablespoons (60g) almond butter
- 1 teaspoon ground cinnamon
- Optional: Drizzle of maple syrup or honey for sweetness

INSTRUCTIONS:

1. Wash and slice the apple into thin wedges or rounds.
2. Take each apple slice and spread a thin layer of almond butter on one side.
3. Arrange the almond butter-covered apple slices on a plate.
4. Sprinkle ground cinnamon evenly over the apple slices.
5. If desired, sprinkle a little honey or maple syrup over the apple slices to give them more sweetness.

Nutritional Information (per serving):

Calories: 436 | Fat: 19g | Saturated Fat: 1.6g | Cholesterol: 0mg | Sodium: 9mg | Carbohydrate: 77.1g | Fiber: 35.2g | Protein: 9.4g

NOTES:

- Customize by using your favorite apple variety and adjusting the thickness of the slices.
- Experiment with different nut butter for flavor variety.

7.5 Cottage Cheese and Pineapple Kabobs

Preparation time	Cooking time	Servings
15 minutes	-	2

INGREDIENTS:

- 2 cups (480g) cottage cheese
- 2 cups (400g) fresh pineapple, cut into bite-sized chunks
- Wooden or metal skewers

INSTRUCTIONS:

1. To keep wooden skewers from burning when cooking, soak them in water for around half an hour.
2. Thread alternating cottage cheese and pineapple pieces onto the skewers, creating colorful and tasty kabobs.

Nutritional Information (per serving):

Calories: 140 | Fat: 2.1g | Saturated Fat: 1.2g | Cholesterol: 8mg | Sodium: 407mg | Carbohydrate: 16.8g | Fiber: 1.4g | Protein: 14.3g

NOTES:

- Experiment with other fruits like strawberries or melons for variety.
- If desired, drizzle with honey for extra sweetness.

7.6 Spiced Roasted Chickpeas

Preparation time	Cooking time	Servings
10 minutes	25 minutes	2

INGREDIENTS:

- 2 cups (480g) canned chickpeas, drained and rinsed
- 2 tablespoons (30ml) olive oil
- 1 teaspoon ground cumin
- 1 teaspoon smoked paprika
- 1/2 teaspoon ground coriander
- 1/2 teaspoon garlic powder
- 1/2 teaspoon onion powder
- 1/2 teaspoon cayenne pepper (change the amount of spice according to taste)
- To taste, add salt and pepper.

INSTRUCTIONS:

1. Preheat your oven to 400°F (200°C).
2. Pat the canned chickpeas dry using a paper towel. Removing excess moisture helps achieve crispiness.
3. Chickpeas should be in a bowl with olive oil, cayenne pepper, smoked paprika, ground coriander, garlic powder, onion powder, and ground cumin. Toss until the chickpeas are well coated.
4. Arrange the spiced chickpeas in a single layer on a parchment paper-lined baking sheet.
5. Cook the chickpeas for 20 to 25 minutes in a preheated oven or until they are crispy and golden brown. Shake the pan or stir the chickpeas halfway through the cooking time for even roasting.

Nutritional Information (per serving):

Calories: 1879 | Fat: 123.5g | Saturated Fat: 17.2g | Cholesterol: 0mg | Sodium: 186mg | Carbohydrate: 196.5g | Fiber: 66g | Protein: 51.3g

NOTES: Experiment with your favorite spices to create different flavor profiles.

_____
_____
_____
_____

7.7 Dark Chocolate-Dipped Strawberries

Preparation time	Cooking time	Servings
20 minutes	5 minutes	2

INGREDIENTS:

- 1 cup (about 175g) dark chocolate chips or chopped dark chocolate
- 1 pint (about 300g) fresh strawberries, washed and dried

INSTRUCTIONS:

1. Ensure the strawberries are thoroughly washed and dried. This helps the chocolate adhere better.
2. Apply a double boiler or microwave to a heatproof bowl to melt the dark chocolate. If using a microwave, heat in 20-second intervals, stirring in between until smooth.
3. Every strawberry should be held by its stem as you dip it into the molten dark chocolate, covering roughly two-thirds of the fruit.
4. Place the dipped strawberries on a parchment paper-lined tray, ensuring they are not touching each other.
5. Place the tray in the refrigerator for at least 30 minutes or until the chocolate is set.

Nutritional Information (per serving):

Calories: 249 | Fat: 13.5g | Saturated Fat: 8.3g | Cholesterol: 0mg | Sodium: 1mg | Carbohydrate: 37.2g | Fiber: 1g | Protein: 3.7g

NOTES:

- Experiment with different types of dark chocolate for varied flavor profiles.
- Optionally, sprinkle chopped nuts or shredded coconut on the chocolate before it sets for added texture.

_____
_____
_____
_____

7.8 Avocado and Tomato Salsa

Preparation time	Cooking time	Servings
10 minutes	-	2

INGREDIENTS:

- 1 large avocado, diced
- 1 cup (about 200g) cherry tomatoes, quartered
- 1/4 cup (15g) red onion, finely chopped
- 1/4 cup (15g) fresh cilantro, chopped
- 1 lime, juiced
- 1 tablespoon (15ml) extra-virgin olive oil
- Salt and pepper, to taste
- Optional: 1 jalapeño, finely chopped (for added heat)

INSTRUCTIONS:

1. Chop the fresh cilantro, finely chop the red onion, dice the avocado, and quarter the cherry tomatoes.
2. Gently combine the diced avocado, quartered cherry tomatoes, chopped red onion, and cilantro in a bowl.
3. Pour the extra virgin olive oil and lime juice over the avocado and tomato combination. Toss gently to coat.
4. Season the salsa with salt and pepper to taste. Adjust the seasoning as needed.
5. Add finely sliced jalapeño to the salsa for a little heat. Adapt the amount to your preferred level of spice.
6. Chill (Optional): Allow the salsa to chill in the refrigerator for 15-30 minutes to let the flavors meld.

Nutritional Information (per serving):

Calories: 549 | Fat: 57g | Saturated Fat: 8.8g | Cholesterol: 0mg | Sodium: 19392mg | Carbohydrate: 16.1g | Fiber: 7.4g | Protein: 2.8g

NOTES: Customize with additional ingredients like diced cucumber or black beans for extra texture.

___
___
___
___

7.9 Hummus-Stuffed Mini Bell Peppers

Preparation time	Cooking time	Servings
15 minutes	10-12 minutes	4

INGREDIENTS:

- 12 mini bell peppers, halved and seeds removed
- 1 cup (240g) hummus (store-bought or homemade)
- 1/4 cup (30g) cherry tomatoes, diced
- 1/4 cup (15g) cucumber, finely diced
- 1/4 cup (40g) red onion, finely chopped
- 2 tablespoons (30ml) extra-virgin olive oil
- 1 tablespoon (15ml) balsamic glaze
- Fresh parsley, chopped, for garnish
- To taste, add salt and pepper.

INSTRUCTIONS:

1. Preheat the oven to 375°F (190°C).
2. Place the mini bell peppers, cut side up, on a baking sheet.
3. Mix the hummus, cherry tomatoes, cucumber, and red onion in a bowl. Season with salt and pepper to taste.
4. Spoon the hummus mixture into each mini bell pepper half, evenly distributing the filling.
5. Drizzle extra-virgin olive oil and balsamic glaze over the stuffed peppers.
6. Bake in a preheated oven for 10 to 12 minutes or until the peppers are just beginning to soften.
7. Take it out of the oven and top it with finely chopped fresh parsley.
8. Allow to cool for a few minutes before serving.

Nutritional Information (per serving):

Calories: 538 | Fat: 49.3g | Saturated Fat: 7.1g | Cholesterol: 0mg | Sodium: 118mg | Carbohydrate: 27.9g | Fiber: 8.9g | Protein: 5.9g

NOTES:

- Experiment with different hummus flavors for variety.
- Serve as a delightful appetizer or a colorful addition to your party platter.

CHAPTER 8: SWEET INDULGENCES

These sweet indulgences are crafted to satisfy your sweet tooth while incorporating wholesome ingredients. Enjoy these guilt-free treats!

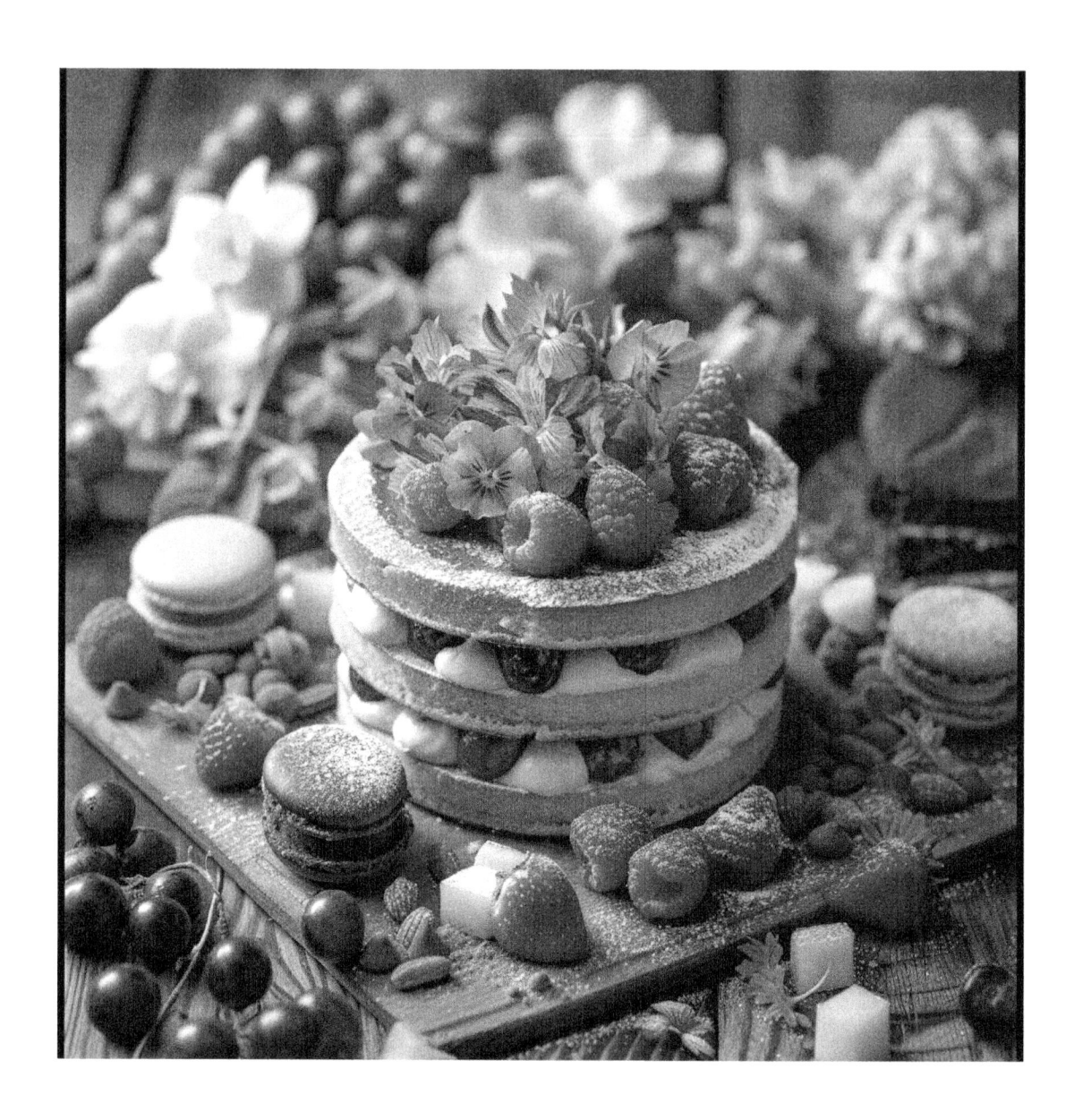

8.1 Dark Chocolate Avocado Mousse

Preparation time	Cooking time	Servings
10 minutes	-	2

INGREDIENTS:

- 2 ripe avocados
- 1/2 cup (50g) unsweetened cocoa powder
- 1/2 cup (120ml) maple syrup or agave nectar
- 1 teaspoon vanilla extract
- A pinch of salt
- 1/4 cup (60ml) coconut milk or any non-dairy milk
- 3.5 oz (100g) dark chocolate, melted and slightly cooled
- Garnish with fresh berries or mint leaves (optional).

INSTRUCTIONS:

1. Transfer the flesh to a food processor or blender once the avocados have been cut in half and the pits removed.
2. Add the agave nectar or maple syrup, coconut milk, vanilla extract, cocoa powder, and salt to the blender.
3. Scrape down the sides as necessary, and blend until the mixture is creamy and smooth.
4. Melt the dark chocolate in a different bowl and allow it to cool a little.
5. Blend the avocado mixture one more after thoroughly blending the melted chocolate.
6. Taste the mousse and adjust sweetness or chocolate intensity if needed.
7. Divide the mousse into two serving glasses or bowls.
8. Chill in the refrigerator for at least 1-2 hours to allow the mousse to set.
9. Before serving, garnish with fresh berries or mint leaves if desired.

Nutritional Information (per serving):

Calories: 1436 | Fat: 77.9g | Saturated Fat: 45.2g | Cholesterol: 40mg | Sodium: 19537mg | Carbohydrate: 149.9g | Fiber: 21.2g | Protein: 20.5g

NOTES:

- Make sure the dark chocolate is slightly cooled to avoid cooking the avocado.
- Experiment with different toppings like chopped nuts or shredded coconut.

_____
_____
_____
_____

8.2 Berry and Yogurt Parfait with Honey Drizzle

Preparation time	Cooking time	Servings
10 minutes	-	2

INGREDIENTS:

- 1 cup (240g) Greek yogurt
- 1 cup mixed berries (strawberries, blueberries, raspberries)
- 2 tablespoons honey
- 1/4 cup (25g) granola
- Fresh mint leaves for garnish (optional)

INSTRUCTIONS:

1. Spoon a layer of Greek yogurt as the base for your parfait in a bowl.
2. Wash and prepare the mixed berries, then add a layer of berries over the yogurt.
3. Drizzle a tablespoon of honey over the berries.
4. Sprinkle a layer of granola on top.
5. Repeat the layers until you reach the top of the serving glass or bowl.
6. Finish with a drizzle of the remaining honey.
7. For extra freshness, you can optionally garnish with fresh mint leaves.

Nutritional Information (per serving):

Calories: 403 | Fat: 4.6g | Saturated Fat: 1.4g | Cholesterol: 3mg | Sodium: 39mg | Carbohydrate: 101.4g | Fiber: 6.9g | Protein: 8.9g

NOTES:

- Customize with your favorite berries or fruits.
- Experiment with flavored yogurts for additional variety.

8.3 Baked Apples with Cinnamon and Walnuts

Preparation time	Cooking time	Servings
15 minutes	20-25 minutes	2

INGREDIENTS:

- 2 large apples (such as Honeycrisp or Granny Smith)
- 2 tablespoons (30g) chopped walnuts
- 2 tablespoons (30g) brown sugar
- 1 teaspoon ground cinnamon
- 1 tablespoon (15g) unsalted butter, melted
- A pinch of salt
- For serving, vanilla ice cream or yogurt (optional)

INSTRUCTIONS:

1. Preheat your oven to 375°F (190°C).
2. Wash and core the apples, removing the seeds and creating a well in the center.
3. Combine the chopped walnuts, brown sugar, ground cinnamon, and some salt in a small bowl.
4. Stuff each apple with the walnut mixture, pressing it gently into the well.
5. The filled apples should be put on a baking dish.
6. Drizzle melted butter over the stuffed apples.
7. Bake for 20 to 25 minutes, or until the apples are soft, in an oven that has been warmed.
8. Once baked, remove from the oven and let them cool slightly.
9. Warm baked apples can be served warm with a dollop of yogurt or vanilla ice cream if desired.

Nutritional Information (per serving):

Calories: 1596 | Fat: 100.6g | Saturated Fat: 29.2g | Cholesterol: 108mg | Sodium: 19704mg | Carbohydrate: 179.1g | Fiber: 38.8g | Protein: 27.2g

NOTES:

- Experiment with different apple varieties for varied flavors.
- You can taste and adjust the sweetness.

_____
_____
_____
_____

8.4 Mango Coconut Chia Pudding

Preparation time	Cooking time	Servings
10 minutes	3 hours (chilling time)	2

INGREDIENTS:

- 1/4 cup (45g) chia seeds
- 1 cup (240ml) coconut milk
- 1 ripe mango, peeled and diced
- 1 tablespoon (15ml) honey or maple syrup (adjust to taste)
- 1/2 teaspoon vanilla extract
- Shredded coconut and additional mango slices for garnish (optional)

INSTRUCTIONS:

1. Combine chia seeds, coconut milk, honey or maple syrup, and vanilla extract in a bowl. Stir well to combine.
2. To prevent clumping, whisk the mixture once more after letting it settle for five minutes.
3. To enable the chia seeds to absorb the liquid and take on the consistency of pudding, cover the bowl and place it in the refrigerator for at least three hours, preferably overnight.
4. Before serving, dice the ripe mango.
5. Once the chia pudding has set, give it a good stir to ensure a smooth texture.
6. Spoon the chia pudding into serving glasses or bowls.
7. For added texture and flavor, top the pudding with diced mango and shredded coconut.
8. If desired, drizzle with more honey or maple syrup.
9. Garnish with additional mango slices.
10. Serve chilled and enjoy the tropical goodness of Mango Coconut Chia Pudding!

Nutritional Information (per serving):

Calories: 607 | Fat: 32.7g | Saturated Fat: 25.8g | Cholesterol: 0mg | Sodium: 24mg | Carbohydrate: 67.5g | Fiber: 10.8g | Protein: 5.5g

NOTES:

- Change the sweetness to your liking by adding more or less honey or maple syrup.
- Experiment with other fruits or nuts for variety.

_____
_____
_____
_____

8.5 Banana-Oatmeal Cookies with Raisins

Preparation time	Cooking time	Servings
10 minutes	12-15 minutes	2 (about 8 cookies)

INGREDIENTS:

- 2 ripe bananas, mashed
- 1 cup (90g) rolled oats
- 1/4 cup (60g) raisins
- 1/4 cup (60g) unsweetened applesauce
- 1/2 teaspoon ground cinnamon
- 1/2 teaspoon vanilla extract
- Pinch of salt
- Optional: 1/4 cup (30g) chopped nuts (walnuts or almonds)

INSTRUCTIONS:

1. Preheat the oven to 350°F (180°C).
2. Combine mashed bananas, rolled oats, raisins, applesauce, ground cinnamon, vanilla extract, and a pinch of salt in a mixing bowl. Mix well.
3. If desired, fold in chopped nuts for added crunch and flavor.
4. Drop cookie-sized portions onto the prepared baking sheet using a spoon, leaving space between each.
5. Using the spoon's back, gently flatten each biscuit.
6. Bake in a preheated oven for 12 to 15 minutes or until the edges start to brown.

Nutritional Information (per serving):

Calories: 529 | Fat: 10.4g | Saturated Fat: 1.6g | Cholesterol: 0mg | Sodium: 19473mg | Carbohydrate: 94.5g | Fiber: 22.7g | Protein: 11.3g

NOTES:

- Experiment with adding chocolate chips or dried fruit for different flavor variations.
- Adjust sweetness by adding more raisins or a touch of honey if desired.

_____
_____
_____
_____

8.6 Almond Butter Banana Ice Cream

Preparation time	Freezing Time	Servings
5 minutes	2-3 hours	2

INGREDIENTS:

- 3 ripe bananas, sliced and frozen
- 2 tablespoons (30g) almond butter
- 1/2 teaspoon vanilla extract
- Optional toppings: sliced almonds, dark chocolate chips, or a drizzle of honey

INSTRUCTIONS:

1. Peel and slice the ripe bananas. Arrange the banana slices on a tray or plate coated with parchment paper in a single layer.
2. Slices of banana should be frozen for two to three hours or until solid.
3. After the banana slices are frozen, put them in a food processor or blender.
4. Add almond butter and vanilla extract to the blender.
5. The ingredients should be blended until smooth and creamy, scraping down the sides as needed.
6. To aid in mixing, add a small amount of almond milk if the mixture is too thick.
7. Once in a bowl, transfer the ice cream and stir in more chopped almonds or dark chocolate chips, if preferred.
8. Serve the Almond Butter Banana Ice Cream immediately for a soft-serve consistency, or freeze for 30 minutes for a firmer texture.
9. Top with sliced almonds, dark chocolate chips, or a drizzle of honey before serving.

Nutritional Information (per serving):

Calories: 384 | Fat: 16.5g | Saturated Fat: 1.4g | Cholesterol: 0mg | Sodium: 5mg | Carbohydrate: 43.4g | Fiber: 7g | Protein: 8.1g

NOTES:

- Experiment with different nut butter for varied flavors.
- Personalize with your preferred toppings, like shredded coconut or fresh berries.

_____
_____
_____
_____

8.7 Greek Yogurt Berry Popsicles

Preparation time	Freezing Time	Servings
10 minutes	4-6 hours	2

INGREDIENTS:

- 1 cup (240g) Greek yogurt
- 1 cup (150g) mixed berries (strawberries, blueberries, raspberries)
- 2 tablespoons (30ml) honey or maple syrup
- 1/2 teaspoon vanilla extract

INSTRUCTIONS:

1. Blend Greek yogurt, honey (or maple syrup), and vanilla extract in a bowl.
2. Wash and prepare the mixed berries. If using strawberries, hull and slice them into smaller pieces.
3. Gently fold the mixed berries into the Greek yogurt mixture, ensuring even distribution.
4. After spooning the mixture into the popsicle molds, gently tap them on the counter to eliminate any trapped air.
5. Make sure the popsicle sticks are firmly inserted into the center of each mold.
6. The popsicles should be frozen for at least four to six hours or until frozen through.
7. To release the popsicles from the molds once frozen, briefly run them under warm water.

Nutritional Information (per serving):

Calories: 439 | Fat: 1.2g | Saturated Fat: 0.8g | Cholesterol: 3mg | Sodium: 23mg | Carbohydrate: 93.7g | Fiber: 2.3g | Protein: 5.4g

NOTES:

- Experiment with different berry combinations for a burst of flavors.
- For added texture, you can sprinkle a layer of granola into each mold before adding the yogurt mixture.

8.8 Chocolate-Dipped Strawberries with Pistachios

Preparation time	Chilling Time	Servings
15 minutes	30 minutes	2

INGREDIENTS:

- 1 cup (about 150g) fresh strawberries, washed and dried
- 1/2 cup (90g) dark chocolate, chopped
- 2 tablespoons (30g) pistachios, finely chopped

INSTRUCTIONS:

1. Prepare a baking sheet or plate lined with parchment paper.
2. Melt the dark chocolate in 20-second bursts in a microwave-safe bowl, stirring in between to ensure smoothness.
3. Make sure the chocolate is melted evenly by holding each strawberry by its stem and dipping it in.
4. After letting any extra chocolate drip off, place the strawberry dipped onto the prepared parchment paper.
5. Immediately sprinkle the finely chopped pistachios over the chocolate-covered part of the strawberry.
6. Repeat the process with the remaining strawberries.
7. Place the chocolate-dipped strawberries in the refrigerator for at least 30 minutes to allow the chocolate to set.
8. Once the chocolate is firm, transfer the strawberries to a serving plate and enjoy this delightful and indulgent treat!

Nutritional Information (per serving):

Calories: 683 | Fat: 54.3g | Saturated Fat: 10.2g | Cholesterol: 6mg | Sodium: 554mg | Carbohydrate: 45.4g | Fiber: 11.9g | Protein: 22.3g

NOTES:

- You can get creative with toppings—try shredded coconut, crushed almonds, or a drizzle of white chocolate.
- Serve the chocolate-dipped strawberries immediately for the best taste and texture.

_____
_____
_____
_____

8.9 Raspberry Lemon Sorbet

Preparation time	Freezing Time	Servings
15 minutes	4-6 hours	2

INGREDIENTS:

- 2 cups (about 300g) fresh or frozen raspberries
- 1/2 cup (120ml) freshly squeezed lemon juice (approximately 2-3 lemons)
- 1/2 cup (120ml) water
- 1/2 cup (120g) granulated sugar
- Zest of 1 lemon

INSTRUCTIONS:

1. Place water and powdered sugar in a small saucepan and heat over medium heat. Stirring causes the sugar to dissolve and form a simple syrup. Remove from heat and let it cool.
2. Put the cooled simple syrup, freshly squeezed lemon juice, and frozen or fresh raspberries in a blender. Blend until smooth.
3. After removing the seeds from the raspberry mixture using a fine-mesh sieve, transfer the smooth sorbet base to a bowl.
4. Add the lemon zest to the sorbet base and stir to incorporate.
5. Transfer the blend into an ice cream machine and process it according to the manufacturer's directions until it attains a consistency similar to sorbet.
6. To firm up, transfer the sorbet to an airtight container and freeze for two to four hours.

Nutritional Information (per serving):

Calories: 268 | Fat: 0.4g | Saturated Fat: 0.2g | Cholesterol: 0mg | Sodium: 7mg | Carbohydrate: 67.7g | Fiber: 4.5g | Protein: 0.9g

NOTES: For a quicker sorbet, you can serve it directly after churning without additional freezing.

_____
_____
_____
_____

8.10 Pumpkin Spice Energy Bites

Preparation time	Chilling Time	Servings
15 minutes	30 minutes	2 (about 10-12 bites)

INGREDIENTS:

- 1 cup (90g) rolled oats
- 1/2 cup (125g) pumpkin puree
- 1/4 cup (60ml) honey
- 1/4 cup (40g) ground flaxseeds
- 1/4 cup (30g) chopped pecans
- 1 teaspoon pumpkin spice blend
- 1/2 teaspoon vanilla extract
- A pinch of salt

INSTRUCTIONS:

1. Rolling oats, pumpkin puree, honey, ground flaxseeds, chopped pecans, pumpkin spice blend, vanilla essence, and a dash of salt should all be combined in a big mixing bowl.
2. Mix the ingredients thoroughly until well combined.
3. Place the mixture in the refrigerator for 15-20 minutes to firm up, making it easier to shape into bites.
4. Once chilled, divide the mixture into small amounts and use your hands to roll them into bite-sized balls.
5. Arrange the Pumpkin Spice Energy Bites on a parchment-lined tray.
6. Place the tray in the refrigerator for 15-20 minutes to set.
7. Once the energy bites are firm, transfer them to an airtight container for storage.

Nutritional Information (per serving):

Calories: 482 | Fat: 16.2g | Saturated Fat: 2g | Cholesterol: 1mg | Sodium: 19415mg | Carbohydrate: 59.2g | Fiber: 10.7g | Protein: 11.6g

NOTES:

- You can add shredded coconut, micro chocolate chips, or chia seeds to make it your own.
- Adjust honey or sweetness according to your preference.

_____
_____
_____
_____

CHAPTER 9: HYDRATION STATION

These beverages are designed to keep you well-hydrated and tantalize your taste buds with a symphony of flavors. Enjoy the refreshing journey at the Hydration Station!

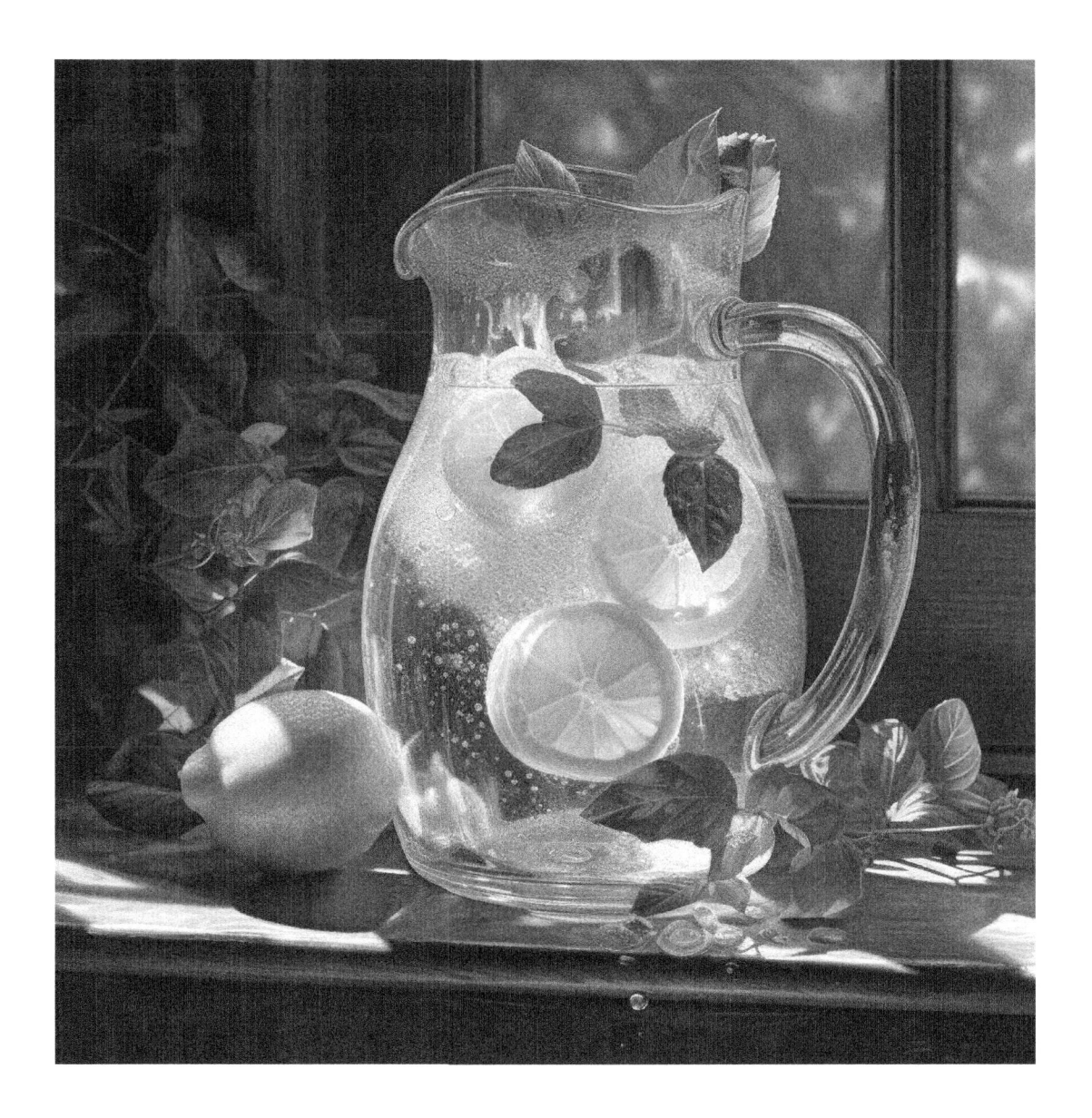

9.1 Citrus Burst Infused Water

Preparation time	Cooking time	Servings
5 minutes	-	2 (about 32 ounces)

INGREDIENTS:

- 2 cups (480ml) cold water
- 1/2 lemon, sliced
- 1/2 lime, sliced
- 1/2 orange, sliced
- 1/2 grapefruit, sliced
- 6-8 fresh mint leaves
- Ice cubes (optional)

INSTRUCTIONS:

1. In a large pitcher, combine 2 cups of cold water.
2. Wash and slice the lemon, lime, orange, and grapefruit into thin rounds.
3. Add the sliced citrus fruits to the water in the pitcher.
4. Tear up some fresh mint leaves and add them to the water for a pleasant taste.
5. Pour ice cubes into the pitcher if you'd like a cold infusion.
6. Stir the ingredients gently to mix them.
7. Allow the Citrus Burst Infused Water to sit in the refrigerator for at least 1-2 hours to let the flavors infuse.

Nutritional Information (per serving):

Calories: 167 | Fat: 2.4g | Saturated Fat: 0.6g | Cholesterol: 0mg | Sodium: 94mg | Carbohydrate: 35.2g | Fiber: 22.7g | Protein: 10.7g

NOTES:

- By allowing the water to infuse for a longer period, you may control the taste intensity.
- Experiment with other citrus fruits like tangerines or blood oranges for variety.

_____
_____
_____
_____

9.2 Berry Bliss Hydration Elixir

Preparation time	Cooking time	Servings
5 minutes	-	2 (about 24 ounces)

INGREDIENTS:

- 1 cup (240ml) cold water
- 1/2 cup (120ml) coconut water
- 1/2 cup (75g) mixed berries (blueberries, raspberries, strawberries)
- 1 tablespoon (15ml) honey
- 1/2 lemon, juiced
- Ice cubes (optional)
- Fresh mint leaves for garnish

INSTRUCTIONS:

1. Blend 1 cup cold water and 1/2 cup coconut water in a blender.
2. Add the mixed berries (blueberries, raspberries, strawberries) to the blender.
3. Squeeze the juice of half a lemon into the blender.
4. Drizzle 1 tablespoon of honey into the mix for natural sweetness.
5. Blend the ingredients until smooth.
6. If desired, strain the mixture to remove berry seeds for a smoother texture.
7. Optional: Add ice cubes to the blender and pulse for a refreshing chill.

Nutritional Information (per serving):

Calories: 177 | Fat: 0.2g | Saturated Fat: 0.1g | Cholesterol: 0mg | Sodium: 30mg | Carbohydrate: 47.5g | Fiber: 2.2g | Protein: 0.6g

NOTES:

- You can add a different amount of honey to get the desired sweetness.
- Feel free to experiment with different berry combinations.

9.3 Minty Cucumber Spa Quencher

Preparation time	Cooking time	Servings
10 minutes	-	2 (about 24 ounces)

INGREDIENTS:

- 1 cup (240ml) cold water
- 1 cucumber, peeled and thinly sliced
- 1/4 cup (15g) fresh mint leaves
- 1 tablespoon (15ml) agave nectar or honey
- 1 lime, thinly sliced
- Ice cubes
- Cucumber rounds and mint sprigs for garnish

INSTRUCTIONS:

1. In a pitcher, combine 1 cup of cold water.
2. Add the thinly sliced cucumber to the pitcher.
3. Tear the new mint leaves and include them in the concoction.
4. Squeeze the juice of one lime into the pitcher.
5. Drizzle 1 tablespoon of agave nectar or honey for sweetness.
6. Stir the ingredients well to infuse the flavors.
7. Refrigerate the spa quencher for at least 30 minutes to enhance the infusion.
8. Incorporate ice cubes into the pitcher before serving.
9. Pour the Minty Cucumber Spa Quencher into glasses.
10. Garnish each glass with cucumber rounds and a sprig of mint.

Nutritional Information (per serving):

Calories: 180 | Fat: 0.3g | Saturated Fat: 0.1g | Cholesterol: 0mg | Sodium: 9mg | Carbohydrate: 49.3g | Fiber: 2.6g | Protein: 1.2g

NOTES:

- Adjust sweetness by adding more or less agave nectar or honey.
- Experiment with different herb-infused waters by trying basil or lemon verbena.

9.4 Green Tea and Berry Fusion

Preparation time	Cooking time	Servings
5 minutes	-	2 (about 16 ounces each)

INGREDIENTS:

- 2 green tea bags
- 2 cups (480ml) boiling water
- 1 cup (150g) mixed berries (strawberries, blueberries, raspberries)
- 1 tablespoon (15ml) honey or agave nectar
- Ice cubes
- Fresh mint leaves for garnish (optional)

INSTRUCTIONS:

1. Place 2 green tea bags in a heatproof pitcher.
2. Over the tea bags, pour 2 cups of boiling water.
3. Allow the tea to steep for 3-5 minutes, depending on your desired strength.
4. When the tea bags are removed, the brewed tea should cool to room temperature.
5. Once cooled, refrigerate the green tea for at least 30 minutes.
6. Mix the agave nectar or honey with the mixed berries in another bowl. Mash lightly to release some of the berry juices.
7. Add the berry mixture to the chilled green tea and stir well.
8. Fill two glasses with ice cubes.
9. Pour the Green Tea and Berry Fusion over the ice.
10. Garnish with fresh mint leaves if desired.
11. Stir gently before sipping to distribute the berry goodness.

Nutritional Information (per serving):

Calories: 177 | Fat: 0.2g | Saturated Fat: 0g | Cholesterol: 0mg | Sodium: 5mg | Carbohydrate: 47.3g | Fiber: 2.2g | Protein: 0.2g

NOTES:

- Add more or less honey or agave nectar to adjust the sweetness.
- Experiment with different berry combinations for varied flavors.

_____
_____
_____
_____

9.5 Watermelon Mint Cooler

Preparation time	Cooking time	Servings
10 minutes	-	2 (about 16 ounces each)

INGREDIENTS:

- 2 cups (about 300g) fresh watermelon, diced
- 1/4 cup (15g) fresh mint leaves
- 2 tablespoons (30ml) lime juice
- 1-2 tablespoons (15-30ml) honey or agave nectar (adjust to taste)
- 2 cups (480ml) cold water
- Ice cubes
- Garnish with watermelon slices and mint sprigs (optional).

INSTRUCTIONS:

1. Put the fresh watermelon, mint leaves, lime juice, honey, or agave nectar in a blender.
2. Blend until smooth and well combined.
3. If preferred, strain the mixture into a pitcher using a fine-mesh screen to remove the pulp.
4. Add cold water to the pitcher and stir to mix the watermelon mint mixture.
5. Add extra honey or agave nectar after tasting to adjust the sweetness if necessary.
6. Chill the Watermelon Mint Cooler in the refrigerator for at least 30 minutes.
7. Fill two glasses with ice cubes.
8. Pour the chilled Watermelon Mint Cooler over the ice.
9. If desired, garnish with watermelon wedges and mint sprigs.

Nutritional Information (per serving):

Calories: 213 | Fat: 0.3g | Saturated Fat: 0.1g | Cholesterol: 0mg | Sodium: 12mg | Carbohydrate: 58.2g | Fiber: 1.8g | Protein: 1.6g

NOTES:

- You can adjust the mint intensity by adding more or less, based on your preference.
- Experiment with different sweeteners for varied flavors.

_____
_____
_____
_____

CHAPTER 10: COOKING BASICS FOR BEGINNERS

These recipes are designed to help beginners master fundamental cooking techniques and build confidence in the kitchen. Enjoy your cooking journey!

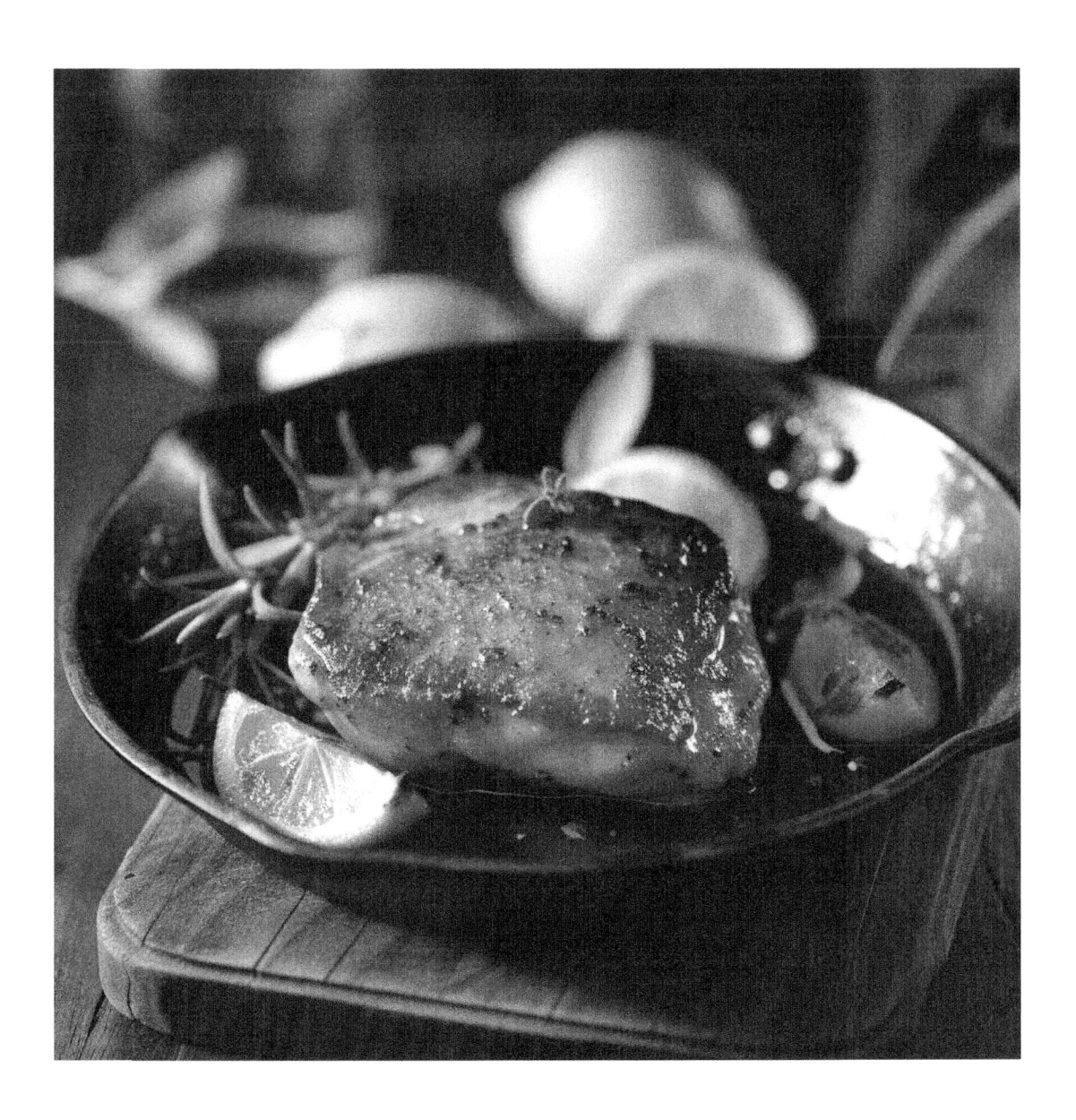

10.1 Easy Pan-Seared Chicken Breast

Preparation time	Cooking time	Servings
10 minutes	15 minutes	2

INGREDIENTS:

- 2 boneless, skinless chicken breasts (about 1 pound or 450g)
- 2 tablespoons (30ml) olive oil
- 1 teaspoon (5g) garlic powder
- 1 teaspoon (5g) onion powder
- 1 teaspoon (2g) dried thyme
- Salt and black pepper, to taste
- Fresh lemon wedges for serving

INSTRUCTIONS:

1. Utilizing paper towels, pat dry the chicken breasts.
2. Combine the dried thyme, onion, garlic powders, salt, and black pepper in a small bowl.
3. Give each side of the chicken breasts an equal coat of the spice mixture.
4. Warm up the olive oil in a big skillet set over medium-high heat.
5. The seasoned chicken breasts should be added to the hot skillet.
6. Sear until golden brown and internal temperature reaches 165°F (74°C), about 6 to 8 minutes per side.
7. After taking the chicken out of the pan, give it some time to rest.
8. Slice the chicken breasts and serve with fresh lemon wedges on the side.

Nutritional Information (per serving):

Calories: 1720 | Fat: 114.8g | Saturated Fat: 19.5g | Cholesterol: 200mg | Sodium: 19641mg | Carbohydrate: 113.3g | Fiber: 27.7g | Protein: 83.7g

NOTES:

- Adjust seasoning according to your taste preferences.
- Use a meat thermometer to ensure the chicken is cooked through but remains moist.

10.2 Simple Spaghetti Bolognese

Preparation time	Cooking time	Servings
15 minutes	15 minutes	2

INGREDIENTS:

- 8 oz (225g) ground beef
- 1 tablespoon (15ml) olive oil
- 1/2 cup (120ml) diced onion
- 1/2 cup (120ml) diced carrots
- 1/2 cup (120ml) diced celery
- 2 cloves garlic, minced
- 1 can (14 oz / 400g) crushed tomatoes
- 1 teaspoon (5g) dried oregano
- 1 teaspoon (5g) dried basil
- Salt and black pepper, to taste
- 2 servings of cooked spaghetti
- Grated Parmesan cheese for garnish
- Fresh basil leaves for garnish (optional)

INSTRUCTIONS:

1. Heat olive oil in a skillet over medium heat.
2. Add diced onions, carrots, celery, and minced garlic. Sauté until vegetables are softened.
3. Add ground beef to the skillet. Using a spoon, break it up and fry till browned.
4. Pour in crushed tomatoes and sprinkle with dried oregano and basil.
5. Season with salt and black pepper. Stir to combine.
6. Lower the heat to low for the sauce to develop flavors, and simmer it for 15 to 20 minutes.
7. While the sauce simmers, cook the spaghetti according to package instructions. Drain.
8. Plate the cooked spaghetti and ladle the Bolognese sauce over the top.

Nutritional Information (per serving):

Calories: 2095 | Fat: 89.1g | Saturated Fat: 24.8g | Cholesterol: 393mg | Sodium: 21520mg | Carbohydrate: 167.1g | Fiber: 54.6g | Protein: 175.8g

NOTES:

- Feel free to customize it with your favorite herbs or add a splash of red wine for extra richness.
- Any leftover sauce can be saved for subsequent use in the refrigerator in an airtight container.

10.3 Roasted Vegetables with Olive Oil and Herbs

Preparation time	Cooking time	Servings
10 minutes	20 minutes	2

INGREDIENTS:

- 2 cups (300g) mixed vegetables (such as carrots, bell peppers, zucchini, and cherry tomatoes), chopped into bite-sized pieces
- 2 tablespoons (30ml) olive oil
- 1 teaspoon (5g) dried thyme
- 1 teaspoon (5g) dried rosemary
- Salt and black pepper, to taste
- 2 cloves garlic, minced
- Fresh parsley, chopped, for garnish

INSTRUCTIONS:

1. Preheat your oven to 425°F (220°C).
2. The chopped mixed vegetables should be combined in a large mixing basin.
3. Drizzle olive oil over the vegetables.
4. Sprinkle dried thyme, dried rosemary, salt, and black pepper. Add minced garlic.
5. Once the oil and seasonings are equally distributed over the veggies, toss them.
6. Arrange the seasoned veggies in a single layer on a baking pan.
7. Roast, tossing occasionally, in the oven for about 20 minutes or until the veggies are soft and beginning to caramelize.
8. Take out of the oven and sprinkle some freshly chopped parsley on top.

Nutritional Information (per serving):

Calories: 1416 | Fat: 107g | Saturated Fat: 19g | Cholesterol: 0mg | Sodium: 316mg | Carbohydrate: 136.6g | Fiber: 59g | Protein: 20.3g

NOTES:

- You can customize the vegetable selection based on your preferences.
- Try varying the flavors by experimenting with herbs such as oregano, thyme, and rosemary.

_____
_____
_____
_____

10.4 Classic Tomato Basil Pasta Sauce

Preparation time	Cooking time	Servings
10 minutes	20 minutes	2

INGREDIENTS:

- 2 cups (500g) canned crushed tomatoes
- 2 tablespoons (30ml) olive oil
- 1/2 cup (75g) onion, finely chopped
- 2 cloves garlic, minced
- 1 teaspoon (5g) dried oregano
- 1 teaspoon (5g) dried basil
- 1/2 teaspoon (3g) sugar
- Salt and black pepper, to taste
- Fresh basil, chopped, for garnish
- Grated Parmesan cheese for serving (optional)

INSTRUCTIONS:

1. Olive oil should be heated in a saucepan over medium heat. Add chopped onion and sauté until translucent.
2. Add minced garlic and sauté for an additional minute until fragrant.
3. Stir in dried oregano and basil, allowing the herbs to bloom in the oil.
4. Add the sugar, black pepper, salt, and smashed tomatoes. Stir well to combine.
5. Bring the sauce to a gentle simmer. Reduce heat to low and let it simmer for about 20 minutes, stirring occasionally.
6. If necessary, taste the sauce and adjust the salt and pepper. If desired, adjust the acidity by adding a small amount of sugar.
7. Just before serving, stir in fresh chopped basil. Optionally, serve with grated Parmesan cheese.

Nutritional Information (per serving):

Calories: 1545 | Fat: 111.7g | Saturated Fat: 22.4g | Cholesterol: 36mg | Sodium: 706mg | Carbohydrate: 136.2g | Fiber: 41.3g | Protein: 37.7g

NOTES: This sauce stays well in the fridge for up to a week in an airtight container. Additionally, it can be frozen for longer preservation.

_____
_____
_____
_____

10.5 Fluffy Scrambled Eggs with Herbs

Preparation time	Cooking time	Servings
5 minutes	5 minutes	2

INGREDIENTS:
- 4 large eggs
- 2 tablespoons (30ml) whole milk
- Salt and black pepper, to taste
- 2 tablespoons (30g) unsalted butter
- 2 tablespoons (8g) fresh chives, chopped
- 2 tablespoons (8g) fresh parsley, chopped

INSTRUCTIONS:
1. Add milk, crack the eggs into a bowl, and season with black pepper and salt. Whisk until well combined.
2. In a nonstick pan set over medium heat, melt the butter. Ensure the entire surface is coated.
3. Pour the whisked eggs into the skillet. Allow them to sit undisturbed, then gently stir with a spatula.
4. Add the chopped parsley and chives as the eggs begin to set. Continue stirring occasionally.
5. Cook the eggs till the doneness you desire. For creamier eggs, remove from heat when they are slightly runny, as they will continue to cook off the heat.
6. Serve the Fluffy Scrambled Eggs with Herbs on toast alongside fresh tomatoes or any other favorite breakfast sides.

Nutritional Information (per serving):
Calories: 1257 | Fat: 107.4g | Saturated Fat: 60.2g | Cholesterol: 969mg | Sodium: 977mg | Carbohydrate: 49.2g | Fiber: 19.1g | Protein: 41g

NOTES:
- Experiment with other fresh herbs like tarragon or chervil for different flavor profiles.
- Feel free to customize it with grated cheese or a splash of cream for extra richness.

10.6 Perfectly Steamed Broccoli

Preparation time	Cooking time	Servings
5 minutes	5-7 minutes	2

INGREDIENTS:

- 1 head of broccoli, washed and cut into florets
- 1 cup (240ml) water
- Salt, to taste
- 1 tablespoon (15ml) olive oil (optional)
- Lemon wedges for serving

INSTRUCTIONS:

1. After giving the broccoli a good wash, cut it into bite-sized florets.
2. Place the broccoli florets in a heatproof colander or a steamer basket.
3. Pour 1 cup (240ml) of water into a pot. Bring it to a boil.
4. Once the water is boiling, place the steamer basket over the pot. Steam the broccoli for five to seven minutes until it is soft but still has a brilliant green color, covered with a lid.
5. After taking the broccoli out of the steamer, place it in a bowl. Season with salt to taste.
6. Drizzle olive oil over the steamed broccoli for added flavor and richness.
7. Squeeze fresh lemon juice over the broccoli for a burst of citrusy freshness.

Nutritional Information (per serving):

Calories: 432 | Fat: 47g | Saturated Fat: 6.7g | Cholesterol: 0mg | Sodium: 19398mg | Carbohydrate: 8g | Fiber: 2.7g | Protein: 2g

NOTES:

- Adjust the steaming time based on your preference for the broccoli's tenderness.
- Customize with additional seasonings like garlic powder or a sprinkle of Parmesan cheese.

_____
_____
_____
_____

10.7 Homemade Chicken Noodle Soup

Preparation time	Cooking time	Servings
10 minutes	**20 minutes**	**2**

INGREDIENTS:

- 1 tablespoon (15ml) olive oil
- 1/2 cup (75g) onion, finely chopped
- 1/2 cup (75g) carrots, sliced
- 1/2 cup (75g) celery, sliced
- 2 cloves garlic, minced
- 4 cups (960ml) chicken broth
- 1/2 teaspoon dried thyme
- 1/2 teaspoon dried oregano
- 1/2 teaspoon dried rosemary
- 1 bay leaf
- 1 cup (60g) egg noodles
- 1 cup (150g) cooked chicken, shredded
- Salt and pepper, to taste
- Fresh parsley, chopped (for garnish)

INSTRUCTIONS:

1. Lightly warm up the olive oil in a pot. Add chopped onions, sliced carrots, and celery. Sauté until vegetables are softened, about 5 minutes.
2. Stir in minced garlic, dried thyme, oregano, dried rosemary, and bay leaf. Sauté for an additional 1-2 minutes until fragrant.
3. Add the chicken broth, reduce the heat, and simmer for ten minutes to let the flavors combine.
4. When the egg noodles are al dente, add them to the pot and cook them as directed on the package.
5. Stir in the cooked and shredded chicken. Simmer the chicken for a further five minutes to fully cook it.
6. Season with salt and pepper to taste. Adjust seasoning as needed.
7. Remove the bay leaf and discard. Warm the homemade chicken noodle soup, sprinkle with fresh parsley, and ladle it into bowls.

Nutritional Information (per serving):

Calories: 1280 | Fat: 65.4g | Saturated Fat: 12.6g | Cholesterol: 53mg | Sodium: 817mg | Carbohydrate: 173.1g | Fiber: 62.9g | Protein: 44.9g

NOTES:

- Feel free to customize with additional vegetables like peas or spinach.
- For a quick option, you can use a rotisserie chicken from the store.

_____
_____
_____
_____

10.8 Basic Baked Salmon Fillets

Preparation time	Cooking time	Servings
10 minutes	15 minutes	2

INGREDIENTS:

- 2 salmon fillets (about 6 ounces/170g each)
- 1 tablespoon (15ml) olive oil
- 1 tablespoon (15ml) lemon juice
- 1 teaspoon dried dill
- 1 teaspoon garlic powder
- Salt and pepper, to taste
- Lemon wedges (for serving)
- Fresh dill, chopped (for garnish)

INSTRUCTIONS:

1. Preheat the oven to 400°F (200°C).
2. Arrange the salmon fillets onto a parchment paper-lined baking sheet.
3. Over the salmon fillets, drizzle some olive oil and lemon juice. Sprinkle dried dill, garlic powder, salt, and pepper evenly.
4. When a fork easily pierces the salmon, it has been baked in a preheated oven for 12 to 15 minutes.
5. Remove the baked salmon from the oven. Serve with lemon wedges on the side and garnish with freshly chopped dill.

Nutritional Information (per serving):

Calories: 1168 | Fat: 55.4g | Saturated Fat: 7.8g | Cholesterol: 174mg | Sodium: 351mg | Carbohydrate: 102.4g | Fiber: 26.6g | Protein: 94.5g

NOTES:

10.9 Creamy Mashed Potatoes

Preparation time	Cooking time	Servings
10 minutes	15 minutes	2

INGREDIENTS:

- 4 medium-sized potatoes (about 2 cups/450g), peeled and diced
- 1/2 cup (120ml) milk
- 2 tablespoons (28g) unsalted butter
- Salt, to taste
- Pepper, to taste
- Chives or parsley chopped (for garnish, optional)

INSTRUCTIONS:

1. In a pot of salted water, add the chopped potatoes. When the potatoes are fork-tender, they are done about 10 to 12 minutes after bringing them to a boil.
2. After cooking, drain the potatoes and put them back in the saucepan.
3. Mash the potatoes using a fork or potato masher to get the consistency you want.
4. Add the unsalted butter and pour in the milk. Continue to mash and mix until the potatoes are creamy and well combined.
5. Season with salt and pepper to taste. Adjust according to your preference.

Nutritional Information (per serving):

Calories: 926 | Fat: 83.4g | Saturated Fat: 52.2g | Cholesterol: 217mg | Sodium: 19995mg | Carbohydrate: 49.4g | Fiber: 15.7g | Protein: 8.8g

NOTES:

- To achieve a creamier texture, vary the quantity of butter or milk used.
- Experiment with variations like adding garlic powder or grated cheese for additional flavor.

10.10 Sautéed Garlic Shrimp

Preparation time	Cooking time	Servings
10 minutes	**5 minutes**	2

INGREDIENTS:

- 1/2 pound (about 225g) large shrimp, peeled and deveined
- 2 tablespoons (30ml) olive oil
- 4 cloves garlic, minced
- 1 tablespoon (15ml) lemon juice
- Salt, to taste
- Black pepper, to taste
- Red pepper flakes (optional for added heat)
- Fresh parsley, chopped (for garnish)

INSTRUCTIONS:

1. Season with salt and black pepper to taste after patting the shrimp dry with a paper towel.
2. Lightly warm up some olive oil in a pan. Add minced garlic and sauté for about 1 minute until fragrant.
3. Add the seasoned shrimp to the pan. Cook for 2-3 minutes on each side until they turn pink and opaque.
4. Quickly toss the shrimp after adding a squeeze of fresh lemon juice.
5. If necessary, add more salt for seasoning, and add red pepper flakes for a little kick of spice. Garnish with chopped fresh parsley.

Nutritional Information (per serving):

Calories: 1435 | Fat: 105.4g | Saturated Fat: 16.1g | Cholesterol: 36mg | Sodium: 19519mg | Carbohydrate: 131.5g | Fiber: 32.9g | Protein: 30.8g

NOTES: You can serve the Sautéed Garlic Shrimp over a bed of pasta or rice or alongside crusty bread to soak up the delicious garlic-infused oil.

CHAPTER 11: CELEBRATING SPECIAL OCCASIONS

These recipes are crafted to elevate your special occasions, creating memorable and delicious moments to cherish. Enjoy the celebrations!

11.1 Elegant Shrimp Cocktail Platter

Preparation time	Cooking time	Servings
15 minutes	5 minutes	2

INGREDIENTS:

- 1/2 pound (about 225g) large shrimp, peeled and deveined, tail-on
- 1 cup (240ml) cocktail sauce
- 1 lemon, sliced for garnish
- Fresh parsley, chopped (for garnish)

INSTRUCTIONS:

1. Cook the shrimp in a kettle of boiling water for 3–4 minutes or until they are opaque and pink. Transfer right away to an ice bath to chill.
2. Prepare the cocktail sauce by combining ketchup, horseradish, Worcestershire sauce, lemon juice, and hot sauce. Adjust quantities to taste.
3. Once the shrimp are cooled, arrange them on a serving platter. You can create a circular pattern or a neat row.
4. Cut a lemon into pieces, then distribute the slices among the shrimp. Sprinkle freshly chopped parsley over the shrimp for a burst of color.

Nutritional Information (per serving):

Calories: 88 | Fat: 0.6g | Saturated Fat: 0.1g | Cholesterol: 36mg | Sodium: 535mg | Carbohydrate: 16.8g | Fiber: 3.1g | Protein: 6.7g

NOTES:

- You can enhance the cocktail sauce with spices like ground black pepper or a dash of celery salt.
- Feel free to customize the garnishes with fresh herbs or microgreens for an extra touch of elegance.

11.2 Herb-Crusted Prime Rib Roast

Preparation time	Cooking time	Servings
15 minutes	1.5 to 2 hours	2

INGREDIENTS:

- 1 bone-in prime rib roast (about 2 pounds or 900g)
- 3 tablespoons (45g) Dijon mustard
- 3 cloves garlic, minced
- 2 tablespoons (30g) fresh rosemary, finely chopped
- 2 tablespoons (30g) fresh thyme, finely chopped
- Salt and black pepper, to taste
- 2 tablespoons (30ml) olive oil

INSTRUCTIONS:

1. Preheat your oven to 450°F (230°C).
2. Using paper towels, pat dry the prime rib roast. Season with salt and black pepper.
3. Mix Dijon mustard, minced garlic, chopped rosemary, chopped thyme, and olive oil to create a herb paste in a bowl.
4. Over the whole surface of the prime rib roast, evenly distribute the herb paste.
5. The roast should be placed bone-side down on a rack inside a roasting pan. To get a good sear, roast in the oven for 15 minutes.
6. Once the internal temperature of the roast achieves the desired doneness (for medium-rare, aim for 135°F or 57°C), lower the oven temperature to 325°F (165°C) and continue roasting.
7. After cooking, take the roast out of the oven and give it 15 to 20 minutes to rest before slicing.

Nutritional Information (per serving):

Calories: 2082 | Fat: 135.5g | Saturated Fat: 28.8g | Cholesterol: 71mg | Sodium: 1902mg | Carbohydrate: 218g | Fiber: 101g | Protein: 64.3g

NOTES: Make sure the roast is cooked to the doneness you desire using a meat thermometer.

___
___
___
___

11.3 Decadent Chocolate Ganache Cake

Preparation time	Cooking time	Servings
15 minutes	**25-30 minutes**	**2**

INGREDIENTS:

For the Chocolate Cake:

- 1/2 cup (60g) all-purpose flour
- 1/4 cup (25g) cocoa powder
- 1/4 teaspoon baking powder
- 1/4 teaspoon baking soda
- Pinch of salt
- 1/4 cup (60ml) vegetable oil
- 1/4 cup (60ml) hot water
- 1/4 cup (50g) granulated sugar
- 1/4 cup (50g) brown sugar
- 1/2 teaspoon vanilla extract
- 1 large egg

For the Chocolate Ganache:

- 1/4 cup (60g) dark chocolate, finely chopped
- 1/4 cup (60ml) heavy cream

INSTRUCTIONS:

Chocolate Cake:

1. Preheat your oven to 350°F (180°C). Grease and flour two 4-inch cake pans.
2. Combine the flour, salt, baking soda, cocoa powder, and baking powder in a bowl.
3. Mix the egg, brown sugar, granulated sugar, vanilla essence, and hot water in a separate basin.
4. Mix until just mixed, then add the dry ingredients to the wet ones. Take caution not to blend too much.
5. Using the prepared cake pans, divide the batter equally. After 25 to 30 minutes of baking, a toothpick inserted in the center should come clean.
6. After 10 minutes of cooling in the pans, move the cakes to a wire rack to finish cooling.

Chocolate Ganache:

1. The heavy cream should be heated in a small saucepan over medium heat until it simmers.
2. Put the dark chocolate, chopped finely, into a heatproof bowl. Pour the hot cream over the chocolate and let it sit for 2 minutes.
3. Cream and chocolate should be thoroughly mixed and smooth.
4. Once the cakes are completely cool, pour the chocolate ganache over one cake layer. Place the second layer on top and pour more ganache over the cake.

Nutritional Information (per serving):

Calories: 589 | Fat: 27.8g | Saturated Fat: 10.5g | Cholesterol: 206mg | Sodium: 3525mg | Carbohydrate: 67.9g | Fiber: 5.1g | Protein: 12.4g

NOTES:
- You can customize the cake by adding nuts, berries, or a dollop of whipped cream.
- Adjust the sweetness of the ganache to your liking by adding more or less chocolate.

_____
_____
_____
_____

11.10 Smoked Salmon and Caviar Canapés

Preparation time 15 minutes	Cooking time -	Servings 2

INGREDIENTS:

- 8 thin slices of baguette
- 2 tablespoons (30g) cream cheese
- 4 oz (115g) smoked salmon
- 2 teaspoons (10g) red onion, finely minced
- 2 teaspoons (10g) capers, drained
- 2 teaspoons (10g) fresh dill, chopped
- 2 teaspoons (10g) chives, finely chopped
- 2 teaspoons (10g) caviar (optional)
- Lemon wedges, for garnish

INSTRUCTIONS:

1. Preheat the oven broiler. Place baguette slices on a baking sheet and toast under the broiler for 1-2 minutes per side or until lightly golden.
2. Put a small amount of cream cheese on each slice of toasted baguette.
3. Place a slice of smoked salmon over the cream cheese on each baguette slice.
4. Sprinkle minced red onion evenly over the smoked salmon.
5. Scatter capers, chopped dill, and chopped chives over the canapés.
6. If using caviar, delicately place a small amount on each canapé.

Nutritional Information (per serving):

Calories: 2352 | Fat: 74.9g | Saturated Fat: 30.5g | Cholesterol: 744mg | Sodium: 11576mg | Carbohydrate: 311.5g | Fiber: 32.4g | Protein: 143g

NOTES: Ensure the baguette slices are toasted just enough to provide a crispy base without being overly hard.

_____
_____
_____
_____

11.4 Sparkling Pomegranate Champagne Punch

Preparation time	Cooking time	Servings
5 minutes	-	2

INGREDIENTS:

- 1 cup (240ml) pomegranate juice
- 1/4 cup (60ml) orange liqueur (such as triple sec)
- 1 tablespoon (15ml) fresh lime juice
- 1 tablespoon (15ml) simple syrup
- 1/2 cup (120ml) chilled sparkling water
- 1/2 cup (120ml) chilled champagne or sparkling wine
- Pomegranate seeds and lime slices for garnish
- Ice cubes

INSTRUCTIONS:

1. Add water and sugar in equal amounts to a small pot. Stir the sugar while heating over medium heat until it melts. Once cooled, you will have simple syrup.
2. Combine pomegranate juice, orange liqueur, fresh lime juice, and simple syrup in a pitcher.
3. Add the chilled sparkling water before serving, and gently swirl to mix.
4. After adding ice cubes to two glasses, evenly divide the pomegranate mixture between them.
5. Pour the chilled sparkling wine or champagne into each glass gradually to combine with the other ingredients.
6. Garnish the drinks with pomegranate seeds and slices of lime.
7. Stir gently and enjoy the refreshing Sparkling Pomegranate Champagne Punch!

Nutritional Information (per serving):

Calories: 251 | Fat: 0g | Saturated Fat: 0g | Cholesterol: 0mg | Sodium: 39mg | Carbohydrate: 54.6g | Fiber: 0.2g | Protein: 0.2g

NOTES:

- Adjust the sweetness by adding more or less simple syrup according to your preference.
- You can rim the glasses with sugar before serving for an extra festive touch.

11.5 Lobster Tail Thermidor

Preparation time	Cooking time	Servings
15 minutes	20 minutes	2

INGREDIENTS:

- 2 lobster tails (about 8 oz each), thawed if frozen
- 2 tablespoons (30g) unsalted butter
- 2 tablespoons (15g) all-purpose flour
- 1 cup (240ml) whole milk
- 1/4 cup (60ml) dry white wine
- 1/4 cup (25g) grated Gruyere cheese
- 1/4 cup (25g) grated Parmesan cheese
- 1 teaspoon Dijon mustard
- 2 tablespoons (30ml) brandy or cognac
- Salt and black pepper, to taste
- Fresh parsley, chopped, for garnish
- Lemon wedges for serving

INSTRUCTIONS:

1. Preheat the oven to 400°F (200°C). Cut through each lobster tail's outer shell using kitchen shears, stopping at the tail fan. Carefully lift the meat, leave it attached at the base, and place it on the shell.
2. Put the lobster tails in a baking sheet arrangement. Bake for about 10-12 minutes or until the lobster meat is opaque and cooked through. Remove from the oven and set aside.
3. In a saucepan, melt butter over medium heat. To make a roux, stir in the flour. Gradually whisk in the milk and wine, ensuring there are no lumps. Cook until the mixture thickens.
4. Reduce heat and add Gruyere and Parmesan cheeses, Dijon mustard, brandy or cognac, salt, and black pepper. To achieve a smooth sauce and melted cheeses, stir.
5. Remove lobster meat from the shells and roughly chop. Fold the lobster into the cheese sauce, ensuring it's well-coated.
6. Preheat the broiler. Spoon the lobster mixture back into the lobster shells. Place under the broiler for 2-3 minutes or until the tops are golden and bubbly.
7. Take it out of the oven, top it with parsley that has been cut, and serve it right away with lemon wedges on the side.

Nutritional Information (per serving):

Calories: 1972 | Fat: 97.8g | Saturated Fat: 58.1g | Cholesterol: 826mg | Sodium: 3318mg | Carbohydrate: 117.7g | Fiber: 19.3g | Protein: 105.7g

NOTES:

_____
_____
_____
_____

11.6 Truffle-Infused Wild Mushroom Risotto

Preparation time	Cooking time	Servings
10 minutes	25-30 minutes	2

INGREDIENTS:

- 1 cup (150g) mixed wild mushrooms (such as shiitake, oyster, or chanterelle), sliced
- 1 cup (200g) Arborio rice
- 1/2 cup (120ml) dry white wine
- 3 cups (720ml) vegetable or chicken broth, kept warm
- 1/2 cup (120ml) heavy cream
- 1/4 cup (60ml) truffle oil
- 1/2 cup (50g) Parmesan cheese, grated
- 1/2 cup (120ml) onion, finely chopped
- 2 cloves garlic, minced
- 2 tablespoons (30g) unsalted butter
- Salt and black pepper, to taste
- Fresh parsley, chopped (for garnish)

INSTRUCTIONS:

1. In a large pan, melt 1 tablespoon of butter over medium heat. Add chopped onions and minced garlic. Sauté until onions are translucent.
2. Add sliced wild mushrooms and cook until they release moisture and become golden brown. Season with salt and pepper. Set aside.
3. In the same pan, add Arborio rice. Toast for 1-2 minutes until the edges become translucent.
4. When the rice has absorbed most white wine, continue stirring after adding it.
5. Begin adding warm broth, one ladle at a time, stirring frequently. Before adding more liquid, let the previous amount be mostly absorbed. Continue cooking the rice until it is al dente and creamy.
6. Pour in the heavy cream, truffle oil, and grated Parmesan. Stir well until the risotto is creamy and the cheese is melted.
7. Gently fold in the sautéed wild mushrooms, ensuring an even distribution throughout the risotto.
8. For more richness, stir in the remaining tablespoon of butter.
9. Season with additional salt and black pepper if needed. Garnish with freshly chopped parsley.

Nutritional Information (per serving):

Calories: 1518 | Fat: 111.1g | Saturated Fat: 63.3g | Cholesterol: 267mg | Sodium: 1367mg | Carbohydrate: 114.7g | Fiber: 18.9g | Protein: 29.5g

NOTES:

- Keep the broth warm throughout the cooking process for consistent absorption by the rice.
- Adjust the truffle oil quantity according to your preference for its distinct flavor.

11.7 Citrus-Glazed Herb-Roasted Turkey

Preparation time	Cooking time	Servings
15 minutes	1 hour 15 minutes	2

INGREDIENTS:

- 1 turkey breast, bone-in (about 1.5 lbs. or 700g)
- 2 tablespoons (30g) unsalted butter, softened
- 2 cloves garlic, minced
- 1 tablespoon (15ml) olive oil
- 1 tablespoon (15g) mixed dried herbs (rosemary, thyme, sage)
- Zest of 1 orange
- Zest of 1 lemon
- Salt and black pepper, to taste
- 1/2 cup (120ml) chicken broth
- Juice of 1 orange
- Juice of 1 lemon

INSTRUCTIONS:

1. Preheat your oven to 375°F (190°C).
2. Utilizing paper towels, pat the turkey breast dry. Season generously with salt and black pepper.
3. To make herb butter, combine melted butter, minced garlic, olive oil, dried herbs of your choice, orange zest, and lemon zest in a small bowl.
4. Gently lift the skin of the turkey breast and rub the herb butter underneath, ensuring even coverage.
5. Combine the chicken broth, orange juice, and lemon juice in a separate bowl. This will be used for basting.
6. Place the seasoned turkey breast in a roasting pan. Pour half of the citrus glaze over the turkey.
7. Once the oven is warmed, roast the turkey for approximately one hour or until its internal temperature reaches 165°F (74°C). Baste with the remaining citrus glaze every 20 minutes for a flavorful crust.

Nutritional Information (per serving):

Calories: 1525 | Fat: 133.8g | Saturated Fat: 59.9g | Cholesterol: 272mg | Sodium: 747mg | Carbohydrate: 65.6g | Fiber: 15.4g | Protein: 35.2g

NOTES:

- Your turkey breast's size will determine how long it takes to cook.
- You can add additional herbs or citrus zest for more flavor.

11.8 Caramelized Onion and Gruyère Tartlets

Preparation time	Cooking time	Servings
15 minutes	30 minutes	2

INGREDIENTS:

- 1 sheet of puff pastry, thawed
- 2 large onions, thinly sliced
- 2 tablespoons (30g) unsalted butter
- 1 tablespoon (15ml) olive oil
- 1 teaspoon (5g) brown sugar
- 1/2 cup (50g) Gruyère cheese, shredded
- Salt and black pepper, to taste
- Fresh thyme leaves for garnish (optional)

INSTRUCTIONS:

1. Preheat your oven to 375°F (190°C).
2. Roll out the puff pastry sheet on a lightly floured surface. Cut into two equal rectangles and arrange on a parchment paper-lined baking sheet.
3. In a pan, heat butter and olive oil over medium heat. After adding the onions, slice them and simmer for 15 to 20 minutes or until golden brown. Stir in brown sugar during the last few minutes to enhance caramelization. Season with salt and black pepper.
4. Spread the caramelized onions evenly over each puff pastry rectangle, leaving a border around the edges.
5. Sprinkle shredded Gruyère cheese over the caramelized onions.
6. Bake in the oven for approximately 15-20 minutes or until the pastry is golden and the cheese is melted and bubbly.

Nutritional Information (per serving):

Calories: 1888 | Fat: 152.3g | Saturated Fat: 64.7g | Cholesterol: 215mg | Sodium: 768mg | Carbohydrate: 145.4g | Fiber: 34.6g | Protein: 15.7g

NOTES: Experiment with different cheeses for varied flavor profiles.

_____
_____
_____
_____

11.9 Grand Marnier Soufflé with Vanilla Sauce

Preparation time	Cooking time	Servings
20 minutes	20 minutes	2

INGREDIENTS:

For Soufflé:

- 2 tablespoons (30g) unsalted butter, softened (for ramekins)
- 2 tablespoons (15g) granulated sugar (for coating ramekins)
- 2 large eggs, separated
- 3 tablespoons (45g) granulated sugar
- 1 tablespoon (15ml) Grand Marnier liqueur
- 1 teaspoon (5g) orange zest
- 1 tablespoon (8g) all-purpose flour
- 1/4 cup (60ml) whole milk

For Vanilla Sauce:

- 1/2 cup (120ml) whole milk
- 2 tablespoons (25g) granulated sugar
- 1 teaspoon (5ml) vanilla extract
- 1 tablespoon (8g) cornstarch

INSTRUCTIONS:

For Soufflé:

1. Preheat your oven to 375°F (190°C). Place a baking sheet inside to heat.
2. Butter the insides of two ramekins and coat them with granulated sugar, tapping out the excess.
3. In a saucepan, heat milk until warm. After adding the flour, simmer for one to two minutes or until a smooth paste develops. Take it off the fire and let it cool a little.
4. Whisk together egg yolks, sugar, Grand Marnier, and orange zest. Gradually whisk in the milk-flour mixture.
5. Beat the egg whites in a different, clean basin until soft peaks form.
6. Fold the egg whites gently into the yolk mixture. Spoon mixture evenly into ramekins that have been prepared.
7. The ramekins should be placed on the prepared baking sheet. Bake for 15-20 minutes or until the soufflés rise and turn golden brown.

For Vanilla Sauce:

1. Whisk together milk, sugar, vanilla extract, and cornstarch in a saucepan.
2. Cook over medium heat, stirring regularly, until liquid thickens.

Nutritional Information (per serving):

Calories: 2148 | Fat: 103.3g | Saturated Fat: 61.4g | Cholesterol: 628mg | Sodium: 1046mg | Carbohydrate: 248.1g | Fiber: 7.1g | Protein: 31g

NOTES:

- Serve promptly, as soufflés tend to deflate quickly.
- Customize the sauce by adding a hint of orange zest for extra citrusy flavor.

CONCLUSION

As we turn the last pages of the "Heart Healthy Cookbook for Beginners," I want to thank you for coming along for the culinary adventure toward a more flavorful and healthier way of living. Eating healthily and heart-healthy doesn't have to mean sacrificing flavor. In fact, it's a chance to experiment with bright flavors and textures and rediscover the joy of cooking excellent meals.

We've included many dishes in this cookbook, from healthy but tempting sweet treats to robust soups, lean proteins, nutrient-dense sides, and vibrant breakfasts and appetizers. Every meal is prepared with your heart health in mind, focusing on whole, wholesome components that enhance general well-being.

Remember that your kitchen is your haven, where you can create, try new things, and enjoy the results of your hard work. This cookbook is meant to empower you, whether a novice or an experienced cook, to make heart-healthy decisions without sacrificing flavor. I invite you to experiment with, adapt, and customize these dishes to fit your dietary requirements and personal tastes as you continue your culinary travels. There's always space for creativity in the kitchen regarding heart-healthy food, which is a broad field. May every bite bring you happiness, sustenance, and contentment, and may your heart be as full as your plate. Cheers to the delicious adventure ahead of you and your heart health.

Have fun in the kitchen!

Morgan Alexandra

"Thank you for dedicating your time to exploring this book. We genuinely value your thoughts, insights, and feedback. Your unique perspective not only aids fellow readers in determining if this book suits them but also offers invaluable guidance to the author. Every opinion holds significance, and we eagerly anticipate hearing yours."

INDEX

Avocado
- Avocado Sunrise Breakfast Wrap (1.2) - p. 13
- Avocado and Tomato Salsa (7.8) - p. 80

Apple
- Cinnamon Apple Overnight Oats (1.11) - p. 22
- Baked Apples with Cinnamon and Walnuts (8.3) - p. 85

Banana
- Nutty Banana Oat Pancakes (1.1) - p. 12
- Banana-Oatmeal Cookies with Raisins (8.5) - p. 87
- Almond Butter Banana Ice Cream (8.6) - p. 88

Beans
- Quinoa and Fruit Breakfast Parfait (1.4) - p. 15
- Spicy Black Bean and Sweet Potato Soup (3.6) - p. 39

Beet
- Roasted Beet and Goat Cheese Salad with Balsamic Glaze (2.7) - p. 30

Berry
- Chia Seed Pudding with Mixed Berries (1.5) - p. 16
- Greek Yogurt Berry Popsicles (8.7) - p. 89
- Berry and Yogurt Parfait with Honey Drizzle (8.2) - p. 84
- Dark Chocolate-Dipped Strawberries (7.7) - p. 79
- Berry Bliss Hydration Elixir (9.2) - p. 95
- Green Tea and Berry Fusion (9.4) - p. 97

Brussels Sprouts
- Garlic Lemon Roasted Brussels Sprouts (5.1) - p. 54

Cauliflower
- Creamy Cauliflower and Leek Soup (3.5) - p. 38
- Cauliflower and Chickpea Curry (5.8) - p. 61

Chicken
- Grilled Chicken Caesar Salad with Whole-grain Croutons (2.5) - p. 28
- Mediterranean Chicken Skewers with Tzatziki (4.6) - p. 49
- Balsamic Glazed Chicken Thighs (4.8) - p. 51
- Easy Pan-Seared Chicken Breast (10.1) - p. 100
- Homemade Chicken Noodle Soup (10.7) - p. 106

Chickpea
- Moroccan Chickpea Stew with Cilantro Drizzle (3.1) - p. 34
- Spicy Chickpea and Turkey Lettuce Wraps (4.9) - p. 52
- Bulgur and Chickpea Salad with Tahini Dressing (6.8) - p. 71

Chocolate
- Dark Chocolate Avocado Mousse (8.1) - p. 83

- Decadent Chocolate Ganache Cake (11.3) - p. 112

Cucumber
- Minty Cucumber Spa Quencher (9.3) - p. 96

Egg
- Mediterranean Egg Muffins (1.3) - p. 14
- Fluffy Scrambled Eggs with Herbs (10.5) - p. 104

Fruit
- Tropical Mango Coconut Smoothie (1.9) - p. 20
- Mango Coconut Chia Pudding (8.4) - p. 86

Garlic
- Sautéed Garlic Shrimp (10.10) - p. 109

Herbs
- Grilled Lemon Herb Salmon (4.1) - p. 44
- Roasted Vegetables with Olive Oil and Herbs (10.3) - p. 102

Kale
- Kale and Quinoa Power Salad with Lemon Vinaigrette (2.1) - p. 24

Lemon
- Spinach and Orzo Lemon Drop Soup (3.2) - p. 35
- Citrus Bliss Salad with Mixed Greens and Oranges (2.3) - p. 26
- Citrus-Marinated Grilled Shrimp Skewers (4.5) - p. 48
- Citrus Burst Infused Water (9.1) - p. 94

Mango
- Tropical Mango Coconut Smoothie (1.9) - p. 20

Mediterranean
- Mediterranean Egg Muffins (1.3) - p. 14
- Mediterranean Greek Salad with Feta and Kalamata Olives (2.4) - p. 27
- Whole Wheat Mediterranean Pizza with Hummus Base (6.4) - p. 67

Mushroom
- Spinach and Mushroom Quiche with Whole Wheat Crust (5.5) - p. 58
- Truffle-Infused Wild Mushroom Risotto (11.6) - p. 116

Nuts
- Nutty Banana Oat Pancakes (1.1) - p. 12
- Trail Mix with Nuts and Dried Fruit (7.1) - p. 74

Olive Oil
- Roasted Vegetables with Olive Oil and Herbs (10.3) - p. 102

Orange
- Citrus Bliss Salad with Mixed Greens and Oranges (2.3) - p. 26

Quinoa
- Quinoa and Fruit Breakfast Parfait (1.4) - p. 15
- Turkey and Quinoa Stuffed Bell Peppers (4.2) - p. 45

- Quinoa and Kale Stuffed Bell Peppers (5.2) - p. 55
- Quinoa and Black Bean Stuffed Peppers (6.2) - p. 65

Salmon
- Grilled Lemon Herb Salmon (4.1) - p. 44

Soy
- Seared Tuna Steaks with Sesame Soy Glaze (4.4) - p. 47

Spinach
- Spinach and Feta Omelet Roll (1.6) - p. 17
- Lentil and Spinach Delight Soup (3.8) - p. 41
- Spinach and Strawberry Salad with Poppy Seed Dressing (2.9) - p. 32
- Spinach and Mushroom Quiche with Whole Wheat Crust (5.5) - p. 58

Sweet Potato
- Spicy Black Bean and Sweet Potato Soup (3.6) - p. 39
- Sweet Potato and Black Bean Skillet (5.3) - p. 56

Tomato
- Tomato Basil Harmony Soup with Whole Wheat Croutons (3.3) - p. 36
- Classic Tomato Basil Pasta Sauce (10.4) - p. 103

Tuna
- Seared Tuna Steaks with Sesame Soy Glaze (4.4) - p. 47

Turkey
- Turkey and Quinoa Stuffed Bell Peppers (4.2) - p. 45
- Spicy Chickpea and Turkey Lettuce Wraps (4.9) - p. 52

Vegetables
- Roasted Beet and Goat Cheese Salad with Balsamic Glaze (2.7) - p. 30
- Minestrone Medley Soup with Garden Vegetables (3.4) - p. 37
- Brown Rice and Vegetable Stir-Fry (6.3) - p. 66
- Farro Salad with Roasted Vegetables and Feta (6.1) - p. 64
- Roasted Vegetables with Olive Oil and Herbs (10.3) - p. 102

Watermelon
- Watermelon and Feta Salad with Mint (2.6) - p. 29
- Watermelon Mint Cooler (9.5) - p. 98

Whole Grain
- Quinoa and Fruit Breakfast Parfait (1.4) - p. 15
- Whole Wheat Crust (5.5) - p. 58
- Whole-grain Couscous with Lemon and Herbs (6.6) - p. 69
- Whole Wheat Mediterranean Pizza with Hummus Base (6.4) - p. 67

Yogurt
- Greek Yogurt and Honey Granola Bowl (1.8) - p. 19
- Greek Yogurt and Berry Parfait (7.3) - p. 76

Printed in Great Britain
by Amazon